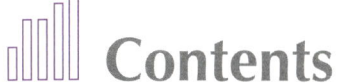 # Contents

On the Web

Health Care Criteria Commentary (https://www.nist.gov/baldrige/baldrige-criteria-commentary-health-care)
- This commentary provides the "why" behind the Health Care Criteria, as well as additional examples and guidance.

About the Baldrige Excellence Framework

The Baldrige framework helps you answer three questions: Is your organization doing as well as it needs to? How do you know? What and how should your organization improve or change?

What can Baldrige do for my organization?

Whether your organization is new, is growing, or has existed for many years, it faces daily and long-term challenges. It also has strengths that have served you well so far. The Baldrige Excellence Framework and its Criteria for Performance Excellence (pages 4–28) incorporate proven practices on current health care leadership and management issues into a set of questions that help you rise to challenges, leverage strengths, and manage all the components of your organization as a unified whole to achieve your mission, ongoing success, and performance excellence. This view of an organization is called a systems perspective.

You may find some of the questions difficult to answer. You may also decide that some questions are not as relevant to your organization as others are. Even so, all the questions will help you identify areas of strength and opportunities to improve your performance and sustainability.

How does Baldrige work?

Baldrige is a nonprescriptive framework that empowers your organization to reach its goals, improve results, and become more competitive. The Core Values and Concepts (see pages 38–43), a set of beliefs and behaviors found in high-performing organizations, are the foundation of the Baldrige framework:

- Systems perspective
- Visionary leadership
- Patient-focused excellence
- Valuing people
- Agility and resilience
- Organizational learning
- Focus on success and innovation
- Management by fact
- Societal contributions and community health
- Ethics and transparency
- Delivering value and results

The Baldrige Criteria are organized into seven categories representing key areas of your organization: (1) Leadership; (2) Strategy; (3) Customers; (4) Measurement, Analysis, and Knowledge Management; (5) Workforce; (6) Operations; and (7) Results. The critical issues facing today's organizations are woven throughout these categories.

I see the Baldrige process as a powerful set of mechanisms for disciplined people engaged in disciplined thought and taking disciplined action to create great organizations that produce exceptional results.

—*Jim Collins, author of* Good to Great: Why Some Companies Make the Leap . . . and Others Don't

Here are some examples of those critical issues.

Resilience and safety. Organizational resilience is the ability to anticipate, prepare for, and recover from disruptions, and to protect and enhance all aspects of your operations when disruptions occur. The Criteria's systems approach prepares you for resilience, and for patient and workforce safety, by helping you understand your organization as a whole, including the changing needs of your organization, staff, physicians, patients, other customers, and stakeholders. Specific questions ask how you reduce and prevent patient harm and how you ensure a safe workplace. The Criteria also ask how leaders intentionally cultivate resilience; how your strategic planning addresses the need for resilience, and how you reinforce resilience in organizing and managing your staff, physicians, and volunteers. Also covered is how you ensure supply-network resilience and organizational continuity and resilience in the event of disasters, emergencies, and other disruptions, taking into account risk, prevention, protection, response, and recovery.

Digitization and technology. Digitization and the use of data analytics, the Internet of Things, artificial intelligence, cloud operations, large dataset-enabled analytics, enhanced automation (including robotics), and other "smart" technologies are accelerating rapidly in health care. The Criteria ask how your leaders consider the need for technological innovation, how your strategic planning considers emerging technologies, how you prepare your staff for changes in technology, and how you incorporate new technology into your health care and business processes. The Criteria also emphasize the use of digital and web-based technologies in patient processes, the need for agility when disruptive technologies arise, and the use of digital data analytics and artificial intelligence in performance analysis and knowledge management.

Innovation. The Criteria lead you to maximize innovation throughout your organization by asking how leaders cultivate intelligent risk taking and innovation; how you incorporate innovation into strategic planning; how you develop priorities for innovation and share information to use in innovation; how you support your workforce in taking intelligent risks; and how you manage, resource, and ultimately decide whether or not to pursue opportunities for innovation.

Diversity, equity, and inclusion. Successful organizations capitalize on the diverse backgrounds and characteristics, knowledge, skills, creativity, and motivation of people, and foster equity and inclusion for all people. The outcome can be improved patient, staff, physician, and stakeholder engagement, as well as improved loyalty and brand image. Questions in the Criteria ask how you ensure fair treatment for your patients and workforce, how you ensure that your workforce represents the diversity in your hiring and patient communities, how you tailor benefits and policies to the diverse needs of your workforce, and how your leaders and your workforce performance management and development foster equity and inclusion.

Cybersecurity. For health care organizations of all kinds, ensuring the security of patient information, as well as managing and reducing cyber risks to other data, information, and operational and other systems, has become a necessity. The Criteria incorporate principles from NIST's *Framework for Improving Critical Infrastructure Cybersecurity*, which focuses on using business drivers to guide cybersecurity activities and considering cybersecurity risks in risk management processes. The Criteria emphasize awareness of emerging security and cybersecurity threats; the role of your workforce, customers, partners, and suppliers in cybersecurity; the importance of identifying and prioritizing information technology and operational systems to secure; and the imperatives of protection, detection, response, and recovery.

Societal responsibility and global sustainability. As the concept of social responsibility has become accepted, high-performing health care organizations see contributing to their community and society as more than something they must do: it can be a driver of customer and workforce engagement and a market differentiator. The Criteria promote societal responsibility and global sustainability through a focus on incorporating societal benefit into strategy and operations, including contributions to supporting and strengthening key communities, protecting the environment, and aiding the social and economic systems around your organization. The Criteria also stress the need to go beyond compliance with relevant laws and regulations.

Other critical issues similarly woven through the Baldrige framework include hiring and retaining a high-performing workforce, capitalizing on your organizational ecosystem, managing enterprise risk, managing for success in a time of rapid change, and many more.

How do I know if Baldrige is right for my organization?

Baldrige is adaptable to any organization's needs. It does not prescribe how you should structure your organization or its operations. In the Organizational Profile (pages 4–6), you describe what is important to your organization. Baldrige encourages you to use creative, adaptive, innovative, and flexible approaches and to choose the tools (e.g., Lean, Six Sigma, International Organization for Standardization [ISO] series, a balanced scorecard, Plan-Do-Check-Act [PDCA]) that are best suited to your organization and are the most effective in driving improvements and sustainable high performance.

How do I know how I'm doing?

With Baldrige, you assess the maturity of your responses based on four evaluation dimensions for the process categories and four for the results category (see the scoring guidelines on pages 32–33).

With the Baldrige framework, you assess and improve your processes along these dimensions:

1. *Approach:* How do you accomplish your organization's work? How systematic and effective are your key approaches?

2. *Deployment:* How consistently are your key approaches used in relevant parts of your organization?

3. *Learning:* How well have you evaluated and improved your key approaches? How well have improvements been shared within your organization? Has new knowledge led to innovation?

4. *Integration:* How well do your approaches reflect your current and future organizational needs? How well are processes and operations harmonized across your organization to achieve key organization-wide goals?

With Baldrige, you assess your results along these dimensions:

1. *Levels:* What is your current performance on a meaningful measurement scale?

2. *Trends:* Are the results improving, staying the same, or getting worse?

3. *Comparisons:* How does your performance compare with that of competitors, or with benchmarks or industry leaders?

4. *Integration:* Are you tracking results that are important to your organization? Are you using the results in decision making?

As you respond to the Criteria questions and assess your responses, you will begin to identify strengths and gaps—first within the Criteria categories and then among them. The coordination of key processes, and feedback between your processes and your results, will lead to cycles of improvement. As you continue to use the framework, you will learn more and more about your organization and begin to define the best ways to build on your strengths, close gaps, and innovate.

What is the impact of Baldrige nationally and globally?

The Baldrige framework and Criteria play three roles in strengthening U.S. competitiveness:

- They help improve organizational processes, capabilities, and results.

- They facilitate the communication and sharing of best practices among U.S. organizations through the Baldrige Award, the Quest for Excellence® Conference, the Baldrige Executive Fellows Program, and other educational offerings.

- They serve as a working tool for understanding and managing organizational performance, guiding your strategic thinking, and providing opportunities to learn.

Baldrige works with public- and private-sector partners to address critical national needs related to long-term success and sustainability, including cybersecurity risk management (see https://www.nist.gov/baldrige/products-services/baldrige-cybersecurity-initiative) and excellence in U.S. communities (see Communities of Excellence 2026, http://www.communitiesofexcellence2026.org).

Within the United States, state, regional, sector, and organizational performance excellence programs use the Baldrige framework to help organizations improve their competitiveness and results. Globally, many performance or business excellence programs use the Baldrige framework or a derivative as their organizational excellence model.

How do I get started?

However you plan to use the Baldrige framework, the Baldrige community is there to help your organization learn, grow, and improve. See the following pages and visit https://www.nist.gov/baldrige to see the possibilities.

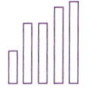 # Health Care Criteria for Performance Excellence Overview and Structure

Health Care Criteria for Performance Excellence Overview: A Systems Perspective

The **performance system** consists of the six categories in the center of the figure. These categories define your processes and the results you achieve.

Performance excellence requires strong **Leadership** and is demonstrated through outstanding **Results.**

The word "**integration**" at the center of the figure shows that all the elements of the system are interrelated.

The **center horizontal arrowheads** show the critical linkage between the leadership triad (on the left) and the results triad (on the right) and the central relationship between the Leadership and Results categories.

The **center vertical arrowheads** point to the Organizational Profile and the system foundation, which provide information on and feedback to key processes and the organizational environment.

The **leadership** triad (**Leadership, Strategy, and Customers**) emphasizes the importance of a leadership focus on strategy and customers.

The **Organizational Profile** sets the context for your organization. It serves as the background for all you do.

The **results** triad (**Workforce, Operations, and Results**) includes your workforce-focused processes, your key operational processes, and the performance results they yield.

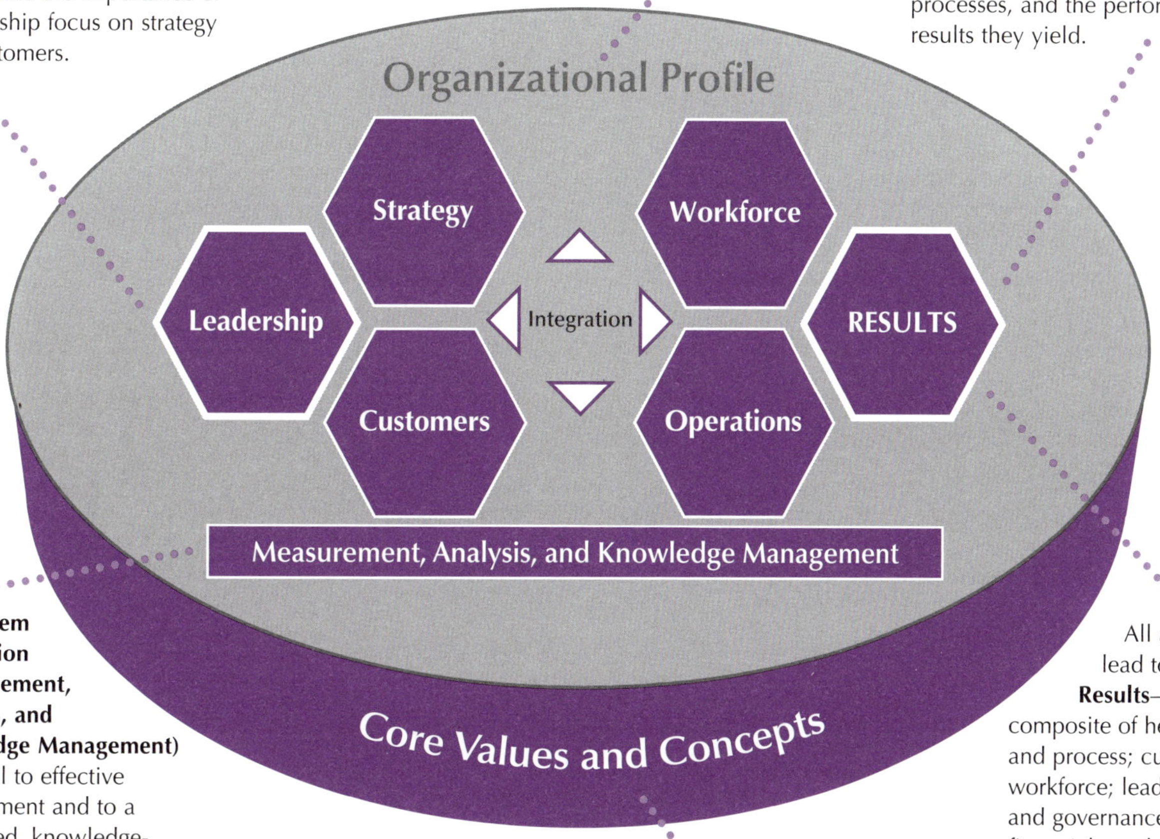

Organizational Profile

Strategy

Workforce

Leadership

Integration

RESULTS

Customers

Operations

Measurement, Analysis, and Knowledge Management

Core Values and Concepts

The **system foundation** (**Measurement, Analysis, and Knowledge Management**) is critical to effective management and to a fact-based, knowledge-driven, agile system for improving performance and competitiveness.

The basis of the Health Care Criteria is a set of **Core Values and Concepts** that are embedded in high-performing organizations (see pages 38–43).

All actions lead to **Results**—a composite of health care and process; customer; workforce; leadership and governance; and financial, market, and strategy results.

Health Care Criteria for Performance Excellence Structure

The seven Baldrige Health Care Criteria for Performance Excellence categories are subdivided into items and areas to address.

Items

There are 17 Health Care Criteria items (plus 2 in the Organizational Profile), each with a particular focus. These items are divided into three groups according to the kinds of information they ask for:

- The Organizational Profile asks you to define your organizational environment.

- Process items (categories 1–6) ask you to define your organization's processes.

- Results items (category 7) ask you to report results for your organization's processes.

See page 3 for a list of item titles and point values.

Item Notes

Item notes (1) clarify terms or questions, (2) give instructions and examples for responding, and (3) indicate key linkages to other items.

Areas to Address

Each item includes one or more areas to address (labeled *a, b, c,* and so on).

Item Questions

Item questions are expressed on three levels:

- *Basic questions* are expressed in the item titles.

- *Overall questions* are expressed in boldface in the shaded box. These leading questions are the starting point for responding.

- *Multiple questions* are the individual ones under each area to address, including the one in boldface. That first question expresses the most important one in that group.

Key Terms

Terms in SMALL CAPS are defined in the Glossary of Key Terms (pages 46–53).

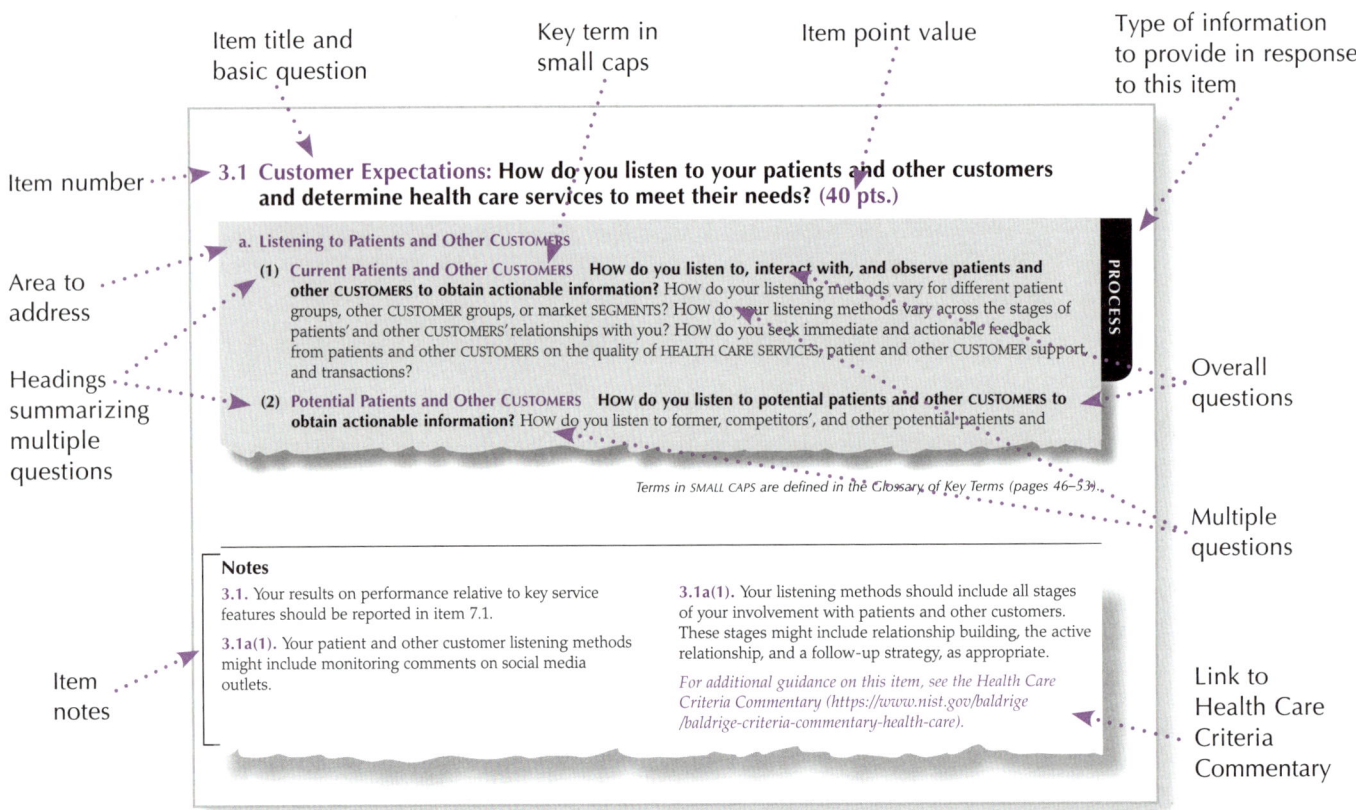

Health Care Criteria for Performance Excellence Items and Point Values

See pages 29–34 for the scoring system used with the Health Care Criteria items in a Baldrige assessment.

P **Organizational Profile**

P.1   Organizational Description

P.2   Organizational Situation

Categories and Items   Point Values

1 **Leadership**   **120**

1.1   Senior Leadership   70

1.2   Governance and Societal Contributions   50

2 **Strategy**   **85**

2.1   Strategy Development   45

2.2   Strategy Implementation   40

3 **Customers**   **85**

3.1   Customer Expectations   40

3.2   Customer Engagement   45

4 **Measurement, Analysis, and Knowledge Management**   **90**

4.1   Measurement, Analysis, and Improvement of Organizational Performance   45

4.2   Information and Knowledge Management   45

5 **Workforce**   **85**

5.1   Workforce Environment   40

5.2   Workforce Engagement   45

6 **Operations**   **85**

6.1   Work Processes   45

6.2   Operational Effectiveness   40

7 **Results**   **450**

7.1   Health Care and Process Results   120

7.2   Customer Results   80

7.3   Workforce Results   80

7.4   Leadership and Governance Results   80

7.5   Financial, Market, and Strategy Results   90

TOTAL POINTS   **1,000**

Health Care Criteria for Performance Excellence

Begin with the Organizational Profile

The Organizational Profile is the most appropriate starting point for self-assessment and for writing an application. It is critically important for the following reasons:

- You can use it as an initial self-assessment. If you identify topics for which conflicting, little, or no information is available, use these topics for action planning.

- It sets the context for understanding your organization and how it operates, and allows you to address unique aspects of your organization in your responses to the Health Care Criteria questions in categories 1–7. Your responses to all other questions in the Criteria should relate to the organizational context you describe in this profile.

- It helps you identify gaps in key information about your organization and focus on key performance requirements and results.

P Organizational Profile

The **Organizational Profile** is a snapshot of your organization and its strategic environment.

P.1 Organizational Description: What are your key organizational characteristics?

a. Organizational Environment

(1) HEALTH CARE SERVICE Offerings   What are your main HEALTH CARE SERVICE offerings (see the note on the next page)? What is the relative importance of each to your success? What mechanisms do you use to deliver your HEALTH CARE SERVICES?

(2) MISSION, VISION, VALUES, and Culture   What are your MISSION, VISION, and VALUES? Other than VALUES, what are the characteristics of your organizational culture? What are your organization's CORE COMPETENCIES, and what is their relationship to your MISSION?

(3) WORKFORCE Profile   What is your WORKFORCE profile? What recent changes have you experienced in WORKFORCE composition or in your needs with regard to your WORKFORCE? What are

- your WORKFORCE or employee groups and SEGMENTS;
- the educational requirements for different employee groups and SEGMENTS;
- the KEY drivers that engage them;
- your organized bargaining units (union representation), if any; and
- your special health and safety requirements, if any?

(4) Assets   What are your major facilities, equipment, technologies, and intellectual property?

(5) Regulatory Environment   What are your KEY applicable occupational health and safety regulations; accreditation, certification, or registration requirements; industry standards; and environmental, financial, and HEALTH CARE SERVICE delivery regulations?

b. Organizational Relationships

(1) Organizational Structure   What are your organizational leadership structure and GOVERNANCE structure? What structures and mechanisms make up your organization's LEADERSHIP SYSTEM? What are the reporting relationships among your GOVERNANCE board, SENIOR LEADERS, and parent organization, as appropriate?

(2) Patients, Other CUSTOMERS, and STAKEHOLDERS   What are your KEY market SEGMENTS, patient and other CUSTOMER groups, and STAKEHOLDER groups, as appropriate? What are their KEY requirements and expectations for your HEALTH CARE SERVICES, patient and other CUSTOMER support services, and operations, including any differences among the groups?

(Continued on the next page)

Terms in SMALL CAPS are defined in the Glossary of Key Terms (pages 46–53).

Notes

P.1a(1). Health care service offerings are the services you offer in the marketplace. Mechanisms for delivering services to your patients or other customers might be direct or might be indirect, through contractors, collaborators, or partners.

P.1a(2). If your organization has a stated purpose as well as a mission, you should include it in your response. Some organizations define a mission and a purpose, and some use the terms interchangeably. Purpose refers to the fundamental reason that the organization exists. Its role is to inspire the organization and guide its setting of values.

P.1a(2). Your values are part of your organization's culture. Other characteristics of your culture might include shared beliefs and norms that contribute to the uniqueness of the environment within your organization.

P.1a(3). Workforce or employee groups and segments (including organized bargaining units) might be based on type of employment or contract-reporting relationship, location (including remote work), tour of duty, work environment, use of flexible work policies, or other factors. Organizations that also rely on volunteers and interns to accomplish their work should include these groups as part of their workforce.

P.1a(5). Industry standards might include industrywide codes of conduct and policy guidance. Depending on the regions and context in which you operate, special financial covenants, standards regarding relationships with physicians or other referral sources, and environmental regulations may apply.

P.1b(1). The Organizational Profile asks for the "what" of your leadership system (its structures and mechanisms). Questions in categories 1 and 5 ask how the system is used.

P.1b(2). Customers include the direct users and potential users of your health care services (patients), as well as referring health care providers and those who pay for your services, such as patients' families, insurers, and other third-party payors. Your organization may use another term for patient, such as client, resident, consumer, or member.

P.1b(2). Patient and other customer groups might be based on common expectations, behaviors, preferences, or profiles. Within a group, there may be segments based on differences, commonalities, or both. You might subdivide your market into segments based on health care service lines or features, service delivery modes, payors, volume, geography, or other defining factors.

P.1b(2). Patient, other customer, stakeholder, and operational requirements and expectations will drive your organization's sensitivity to the risk of service, support, and supply-network interruptions, including those due to natural disasters and other emergencies.

P.1b(3). Your supply network consists of the entities that contribute to producing your health care services and delivering them to your patients and other customers. For some organizations, these entities form a chain, in which one entity directly supplies another. Increasingly, however, these entities are interlinked and exist in interdependent rather than linear relationships. The Health Care Criteria use the term supply network to emphasize the interdependencies among organizations and their suppliers.

For additional guidance on this item, see the Health Care Criteria Commentary (https://www.nist.gov/baldrige/baldrige-criteria-commentary-health-care).

Organizational Profile

5

P.2 Organizational Situation: What is your organization's strategic situation?

a. Competitive Environment

(1) Competitive Position   What are your relative size and growth in the health care industry or the markets you serve? How many and what types of competitors do you have?

(2) Competitiveness Changes   What KEY changes, if any, are affecting your competitive situation, including changes that create opportunities for INNOVATION and collaboration, as appropriate?

(3) Comparative Data   What KEY sources of comparative and competitive data are available from within the health care industry? What KEY sources of comparative data are available from outside the health care industry? What limitations, if any, affect your ability to obtain or use these data?

b. Strategic Context

What are your KEY STRATEGIC CHALLENGES and ADVANTAGES?

c. PERFORMANCE Improvement System

What is your PERFORMANCE improvement system, including your PROCESSES for evaluation and improvement of KEY organizational projects and PROCESSES?

Terms in SMALL CAPS are defined in the Glossary of Key Terms (pages 46–53).

Notes

P.2b. Strategic challenges and advantages might be in the areas of business, operations, societal contributions, and workforce. They might relate to health care services or service features, quality and outcomes, finances, organizational structure and culture, emerging technology, digital integration, data and information security and cybersecurity, emerging competitors, changing stakeholder requirements, workforce capability or capacity, brand recognition and reputation, your supply network, and the health care industry.

P.2c. The Baldrige Scoring System (pages 29–34) uses performance improvement through learning and integration as a factor in assessing the maturity of organizational approaches and their deployment. This question is intended to set an overall context for your approach to performance improvement. The approach you use should be related to your organization's needs. Approaches that are compatible with the overarching systems approach provided by the Baldrige framework might include implementing a Lean Enterprise System, applying Six Sigma methodology, using PDCA methodology, using standards from ISO (e.g., the 9000 or 14000 series, or sector-specific standards), using decision or implementation science, or employing other improvement tools.

For additional guidance on this item, see the Health Care Criteria Commentary (https://www.nist.gov/baldrige /baldrige-criteria-commentary-health-care).

1 Leadership (120 pts.)

The **Leadership** category asks HOW SENIOR LEADERS' personal actions guide and sustain your organization. It also asks about your organization's GOVERNANCE system; HOW your organization fulfills its legal and ethical responsibilities; and HOW it makes societal contributions.

1.1 Senior Leadership: How do your senior leaders lead the organization? (70 pts.)

PROCESS

a. VISION and VALUES

(1) Establishing VISION and VALUES **HOW do SENIOR LEADERS set and DEPLOY your organization's VISION and VALUES?** HOW do SENIOR LEADERS DEPLOY the VISION and VALUES through your LEADERSHIP SYSTEM; to the WORKFORCE; to KEY suppliers and PARTNERS; and to patients, other CUSTOMERS, and other STAKEHOLDERS, as appropriate? HOW do SENIOR LEADERS' personal actions reflect a commitment to those VALUES?

(2) Promoting Legal and ETHICAL BEHAVIOR **HOW do SENIOR LEADERS' personal actions demonstrate their commitment to legal and ETHICAL BEHAVIOR?** HOW do SENIOR LEADERS promote an organizational environment that requires it?

b. Communication

HOW do SENIOR LEADERS communicate with and engage the entire WORKFORCE, KEY PARTNERS, patients, and other KEY CUSTOMERS? HOW do they

- encourage frank, two-way communication;
- communicate KEY decisions and needs for organizational change; and
- take a direct role in motivating the WORKFORCE toward HIGH PERFORMANCE and a patient, other CUSTOMER, and business focus?

c. MISSION and Organizational PERFORMANCE

(1) Creating an Environment for Success **HOW do SENIOR LEADERS create an environment for success now and in the future?** HOW do they

- create an environment for the achievement of your MISSION;
- create and reinforce your organizational culture; a culture that fosters patient, other CUSTOMER, and WORKFORCE ENGAGEMENT, equity, and inclusion; and a culture of patient safety;
- cultivate organizational agility and RESILIENCE, accountability, organizational and individual LEARNING, INNOVATION, and INTELLIGENT RISK taking; and
- participate in succession planning and the development of future organizational leaders?

(2) Creating a Focus on Action **HOW do SENIOR LEADERS create a focus on action that will achieve the organization's MISSION?** HOW do SENIOR LEADERS

- create a focus on action that will improve the organization's PERFORMANCE;
- identify needed actions;
- in setting expectations for organizational PERFORMANCE, include a focus on creating and balancing VALUE for patients, other CUSTOMERS, and other STAKEHOLDERS; and
- demonstrate personal accountability for the organization's actions?

Terms in SMALL CAPS are defined in the Glossary of Key Terms (pages 46–53).

Notes

1.1. In health care organizations with separate administrative/operational and health-care-provider leaders, the term "senior leaders" refers to both sets of leaders and the relationship between them.

1.1. Your organizational performance results should be reported in items 7.1–7.5. Results related to the effectiveness of leadership and the leadership system should be reported in item 7.4.

1.1a(1). Your organization's vision should set the context for the strategic objectives and action plans you describe in items 2.1 and 2.2.

1.1b. Two-way communication may include use of social media, such as delivering periodic messages through internal and external websites, tweets, blogging, and patient and workforce digital forums, as well as monitoring external social media outlets and responding, when appropriate.

1.1b. Senior leaders' direct role in motivating the workforce may include participating in reward and recognition programs.

1.1b. Organizations that rely heavily on volunteers to accomplish their work should also discuss efforts to communicate with and engage the volunteer workforce.

1.1c(1). A successful organization is capable of addressing current organizational needs and, by addressing risk, agility, resilience, and strategic opportunities, of preparing for its future business, market, and operating environment. In creating an environment for success, leaders should consider both external and internal factors. Factors might include risk appetite and tolerance; the need for technological and organizational innovation, including risks and opportunities arising from emerging technology, data integration, and digitization; readiness for disruptions; organizational culture; work systems; the potential need for changes in structure and culture; workforce capability and capacity; resource

availability; societal benefit and social equity; and core competencies.

1.1c(1). Promoting equity means ensuring that all customers and workforce members are treated fairly and that all workforce members can reach their full potential. Inclusion refers to promoting the full participation of all workforce members and ensuring a sense of belonging for them.

1.1c(2). Senior leaders' focus on action considers your strategy, workforce, work systems, and assets. It includes taking intelligent risks, implementing innovations and ongoing improvements in performance and productivity, taking the actions needed to achieve your strategic objectives (see 2.2a[1]), and possibly establishing plans for managing organizational change or responding rapidly to significant new information.

For additional guidance on this item, see the Health Care Criteria Commentary (https://www.nist.gov/baldrige /baldrige-criteria-commentary-health-care).

1.2 Governance and Societal Contributions: **How do you govern your organization and make societal contributions? (50 pts.)**

a. **Organizational GOVERNANCE**

(1) **GOVERNANCE System**   **HOW does your organization ensure responsible GOVERNANCE?** HOW does your GOVERNANCE system review and achieve the following?

- Accountability for SENIOR LEADERS' actions
- Accountability for strategy
- Fiscal accountability
- Accountability for patient safety and health care quality
- Transparency in operations
- Selection of GOVERNANCE board members and disclosure policies for them, as appropriate
- Independence and EFFECTIVENESS of internal and external audits
- Protection of STAKEHOLDER and stockholder interests, as appropriate
- Succession planning for SENIOR LEADERS

(2) **PERFORMANCE Evaluation**   **HOW do you evaluate the PERFORMANCE of your SENIOR LEADERS and your GOVERNANCE board?** HOW do you use PERFORMANCE evaluations in determining executive compensation? HOW do your SENIOR LEADERS and GOVERNANCE board use these PERFORMANCE evaluations to advance their development and improve the effectiveness of leaders, the board, and the LEADERSHIP SYSTEM, as appropriate?

b. **Legal and ETHICAL BEHAVIOR**

(1) **Legal, Regulatory, and Accreditation Compliance**   **HOW do you address current and anticipate future legal, regulatory, and community concerns with your HEALTH CARE SERVICES and operations?** HOW do you

- address any adverse societal impacts of your HEALTH CARE SERVICES and operations,
- anticipate public concerns with your future HEALTH CARE SERVICES and operations, and
- prepare for these impacts and concerns proactively?

What are your KEY compliance PROCESSES, MEASURES, and GOALS for meeting and surpassing regulatory, legal, and accreditation requirements, as appropriate? What are your KEY PROCESSES, MEASURES, and GOALS for addressing risks associated with your HEALTH CARE SERVICES and operations?

(Continued on the next page)

(2) ETHICAL BEHAVIOR   HOW do you promote and ensure ETHICAL BEHAVIOR in all interactions? What are your KEY PROCESSES and MEASURES or INDICATORS for promoting and ensuring ETHICAL BEHAVIOR in your GOVERNANCE structure; throughout your organization; and in interactions with your WORKFORCE, patients, other CUSTOMERS, PARTNERS, suppliers, and other STAKEHOLDERS? HOW do you monitor and respond to breaches of ETHICAL BEHAVIOR?

c. Societal Contributions

(1) Societal Well-Being   HOW do you incorporate societal well-being and benefit into your strategy and daily operations? HOW do you contribute to the well-being of your environmental, social, and economic systems?

(2) Community Support   HOW do you actively support and strengthen your KEY communities? What are your KEY communities? HOW do you identify them and determine areas for organizational involvement? HOW do your SENIOR LEADERS, in concert with your WORKFORCE, contribute to improving these communities and building community health?

Terms in SMALL CAPS are defined in the Glossary of Key Terms (pages 46–53).

Notes

1.2. Societal contributions in areas critical to your ongoing success should also be addressed in Strategy Development (item 2.1) and Operations (category 6). Key societal results should be reported in item 7.4.

1.2a(1). In protecting stakeholder interests, the governance system should consider and approve appropriate levels of risk for the organization, recognizing the need to accept risk as part of running a successful organization.

1.2a(1). The governance board's review of organizational performance and progress, if appropriate, is addressed in 4.1(b).

1.2a(1). Transparency in the operations of your governance system should include your internal controls on governance processes. For some privately held businesses and nonprofit organizations, an external advisory board may provide some or all governance board functions.

1.2a(2). The evaluation of leaders' performance might be supported by peer reviews, formal performance management reviews, reviews by external advisory boards, and formal or informal feedback from and surveys of the workforce and other stakeholders.

1.2b(1). Proactively preparing for adverse societal impacts and concerns may include conserving natural resources, reducing carbon emissions, and using effective supply-network management processes, as appropriate.

1.2b(2). Measures or indicators of ethical behavior might include the percentage of independent board members, instances of ethical conduct or compliance breaches and responses to them, survey results showing workforce perceptions of organizational ethics, ethics hotline use, and results of ethics reviews and audits. Such measures

or indicators might also include evidence that policies, workforce training, and monitoring systems are in place for conflicts of interest; protection and use of sensitive data, information, and knowledge generated through synthesizing and correlating these data; and proper use of funds.

1.2c. Some health care organizations may contribute to society and support their key communities totally through the mission-related activities described in response to other Criteria questions. In such cases, it is appropriate to respond here with any "extra efforts" through which you support these communities.

1.2c(1). Areas of societal well-being and benefit to report are those that go beyond the compliance processes you describe in 1.2b(1). They might include organizational or collaborative efforts to improve the environment; strengthen local community services, education, health, and emergency preparedness; address social inequities; and improve the practices of trade, business, or professional associations.

1.2c(2). Areas for organizational involvement in supporting your key communities might include areas that leverage your core competencies. Actions to build community health are population-based services that support the general health of the communities in which you operate. Such services will likely draw on your core competencies and might include the identification of community health needs, health education programs, immunization programs, health screenings, wellness and prevention programs, indigent care, and programs to eliminate health disparities, perhaps through partnerships with community organizations.

For additional guidance on this item, see the Health Care Criteria Commentary (https://www.nist.gov/baldrige /baldrige-criteria-commentary-health-care).

2 Strategy (85 pts.)

The **Strategy** category asks HOW your organization develops STRATEGIC OBJECTIVES and ACTION PLANS, implements them, changes them if circumstances require, and measures progress.

2.1 Strategy Development: How do you develop your strategy? (45 pts.)

a. Strategy Development PROCESS

(1) Strategic Planning PROCESS   HOW do you conduct your strategic planning? What are the KEY PROCESS steps? Who are the KEY participants? What are your short- and longer-term planning horizons? HOW does your strategic planning PROCESS address the potential need for change, prioritization of change initiatives, and organizational agility and RESILIENCE?

(2) INNOVATION   HOW does your strategy development PROCESS stimulate and incorporate INNOVATION? HOW do you identify STRATEGIC OPPORTUNITIES? HOW do you decide which STRATEGIC OPPORTUNITIES are INTELLIGENT RISKS to pursue? What are your KEY STRATEGIC OPPORTUNITIES?

(3) Strategy Considerations   HOW do you collect and analyze relevant data and develop information for use in your strategic planning PROCESS? In this collection and ANALYSIS, HOW do you include these KEY elements of risk?

- Your STRATEGIC CHALLENGES and STRATEGIC ADVANTAGES
- Potential changes and disruptions in your regulatory and external environment
- Technological changes and INNOVATIONS affecting your HEALTH CARE SERVICES and operations
- Potential blind spots in your strategic planning PROCESS and information
- Your ability to execute the strategic plan

(4) WORK SYSTEMS and CORE COMPETENCIES   HOW do you decide which KEY PROCESSES will be accomplished by your WORKFORCE and which by external suppliers, PARTNERS, and COLLABORATORS? HOW do those decisions consider your STRATEGIC OBJECTIVES; your CORE COMPETENCIES; and the CORE COMPETENCIES of potential suppliers, PARTNERS, and COLLABORATORS? HOW do you determine what future organizational CORE COMPETENCIES and WORK SYSTEMS you will need?

b. STRATEGIC OBJECTIVES

(1) KEY STRATEGIC OBJECTIVES   What are your organization's KEY STRATEGIC OBJECTIVES and their most important related GOALS? What is your timetable for achieving them? What KEY changes, if any, are planned in your HEALTH CARE SERVICES, CUSTOMERS and markets, suppliers and PARTNERS, and operations?

(2) STRATEGIC OBJECTIVE Considerations   HOW do your STRATEGIC OBJECTIVES achieve appropriate balance among varying and potentially competing organizational needs? HOW do your STRATEGIC OBJECTIVES

- address your STRATEGIC CHALLENGES and leverage your CORE COMPETENCIES, STRATEGIC ADVANTAGES, and STRATEGIC OPPORTUNITIES;
- balance short- and longer-term planning horizons; and
- consider and balance the needs of all KEY STAKEHOLDERS?

Terms in SMALL CAPS are defined in the Glossary of Key Terms (pages 46–53).

Notes

2.1. This item deals with your overall organizational strategy, which might include changes in patient and other customer engagement processes and health care service offerings. However, you should describe the patient and other customer engagement and service design strategies, respectively, in items 3.2 and 6.1, as appropriate.

2.1. Strategy development refers to your organization's approach to preparing for the future. In developing your strategy, you should consider your level of acceptable enterprise risk. To make decisions and allocate resources,

you might use various types of forecasts, projections, options, scenarios, knowledge (see 4.2b), analyses, or other approaches to envisioning the future. Strategy development might involve key suppliers, collaborators, partners, patients, and other customers.

2.1. The term "strategy" should be interpreted broadly. Strategy might be built around or lead to any or all of the following: new, changing, or discontinued health care services, including acquisitions or entry into new services to improve access, grow revenue, or reduce costs; redefinition of key patient and other customer groups or market segments; definition or redefinition of your role in your business ecosystem (your network of partners, suppliers, collaborators, competitors, patients, other customers, communities, and other relevant organizations inside and outside the health care sector that serve as potential resources); differentiation of your brand; new core competencies; and new staff or volunteer relationships. It might also be directed toward becoming a high-reliability organization, a provider of a high-end or customized service, an integrated service provider, or an employer of choice, or toward meeting a community or population health care need.

2.1a(1). Organizational agility refers to the capacity for rapid change in strategy and the ability to adjust your operations as opportunities or needs arise.

2.1a(3). Integration of data from all sources to generate strategically relevant information is a key consideration. Data and information might relate to patient, other customer, and market requirements, expectations, opportunities, and risks; financial, societal, ethical, regulatory, technological, security and cybersecurity, and other potential opportunities and risks; your core competencies; the competitive environment and your performance now and in the future relative to competitors and comparable organizations; your culture, policies, and processes to ensure patient safety and avoid medical errors; your clinical outcomes; policies and procedures for access to and equity of care; workforce and other resource needs; your ability to capitalize on diversity and promote equity and inclusion; your ability to prevent and respond to disasters and emergencies; opportunities to redirect resources to higher-priority products, services, or areas; changes in the local or national economy; requirements for and strengths and weaknesses of your partners

and supply network; changes in your parent organization; and other factors unique to your organization.

2.1a(3). Your strategic planning should address your ability to mobilize the necessary resources and knowledge to execute the strategic plan. It should also address your ability to execute contingency plans or, if circumstances require, to shift strategy and rapidly execute new or changed plans.

2.1a(3). Technologies that continue to drive change include enhanced automation, the adoption of cloud operations, the use of data analytics, the Internet of Things, artificial intelligence, and large dataset-enabled business and process modeling.

2.1a(4). Your work systems are the coordinated combination of internal work processes and external resources you need to develop and produce health care services, deliver them to your patients and other customers, and succeed in your marketplace. External resources might include partners, suppliers, collaborators, competitors, customers, and other entities or organizations that are part of your business ecosystem. Decisions about work systems involve protecting intellectual property, capitalizing on core competencies, and mitigating risk.

2.1b(1). Strategic objectives should focus on your specific challenges, advantages, and opportunities—those most important to your ongoing success and to strengthening your overall performance and your success now and in the future.

For additional guidance on this item, see the Health Care Criteria Commentary (https://www.nist.gov/baldrige /baldrige-criteria-commentary-health-care).

2.2 Strategy Implementation: How do you implement your strategy? (40 pts.)

a. ACTION PLAN Development and DEPLOYMENT

(1) ACTION PLANS **What are your key short- and longer-term ACTION PLANS?** What is their relationship to your STRATEGIC OBJECTIVES? HOW do you develop your ACTION PLANS?

(2) ACTION PLAN Implementation **HOW do you DEPLOY your ACTION PLANS?** HOW do you DEPLOY your ACTION PLANS to your WORKFORCE and to KEY suppliers, PARTNERS, and COLLABORATORS, as appropriate, to ensure that you achieve your KEY STRATEGIC OBJECTIVES? HOW do you ensure that you can sustain the KEY outcomes of your ACTION PLANS?

(3) Resource Allocation **HOW do you ensure that financial and other resources are available to support the achievement of your ACTION PLANS while you meet current obligations?** HOW do you allocate these resources to support the plans? HOW do you manage the risks associated with the plans to ensure your financial viability?

(4) WORKFORCE Plans **What are your KEY WORKFORCE plans to support your short- and longer-term STRATEGIC OBJECTIVES and ACTION PLANS?** HOW do the plans address potential impacts on your WORKFORCE members and any potential changes in WORKFORCE CAPABILITY and CAPACITY needs?

(5) PERFORMANCE MEASURES **What KEY PERFORMANCE MEASURES or INDICATORS do you use to track the achievement and EFFECTIVENESS of your ACTION PLANS?** HOW does your overall ACTION PLAN measurement system reinforce organizational ALIGNMENT?

(6) PERFORMANCE PROJECTIONS **For these KEY PERFORMANCE MEASURES or INDICATORS, what are your PERFORMANCE PROJECTIONS for your short- and longer-term planning horizons?** If there are gaps between your projected PERFORMANCE and that of your competitors or organizations offering similar HEALTH CARE SERVICES, HOW do you address them in your ACTION PLANS?

b. ACTION PLAN Modification

HOW do you recognize and respond when circumstances require a shift in ACTION PLANS and rapid execution of new plans?

Terms in SMALL CAPS are defined in the Glossary of Key Terms (pages 46–53).

Notes

2.2. The development and deployment of your strategy and action plans are closely linked to other Health Care Criteria items. The following are examples of key linkages:

- Item 1.1: how your senior leaders set and communicate organizational direction

- Category 3: how you gather patient, other customer, and market knowledge as input to your strategy and action plans and to use in deploying action plans

- Category 4: how you measure and analyze data and manage knowledge to support key information needs, support strategy development, provide an effective basis for performance measurements, and track progress on achieving strategic objectives and action plans

- Category 5: how you meet workforce capability and capacity needs, determine needs and design your workforce learning and development system, and implement workforce-related changes resulting from action plans

- Category 6: how you address changes to your work processes resulting from action plans

- Item 7.1: specific accomplishments relative to your organizational strategy and action plans

- Item 7.5: results for overall strategy and action plan achievement

2.2a(6). Projected performance might consider new ventures; organizational acquisitions or mergers; new value creation; market entry and shifts; new legislative mandates, legal requirements, industry standards, or accreditation standards; and significant anticipated innovations in health care services and technology. Your process for projecting future performance should be reported in 4.1c(1).

2.2b. Circumstances that might require shifts in action plans and rapid execution of new plans include disruptive internal or external events, changes in your competitive environment, changing economic conditions, the emergence of disruptive technologies, and sudden changes in patient and other customer requirements and expectations.

For additional guidance on this item, see the Health Care Criteria Commentary (https://www.nist.gov/baldrige/baldrige-criteria-commentary-health-care).

3 Customers (85 pts.)

The **CUSTOMERS** category asks HOW your organization engages its patients and other CUSTOMERS for ongoing marketplace success, including HOW your organization listens to the VOICE OF THE CUSTOMER, serves and exceeds patients' and other CUSTOMERS' expectations, and builds long-term relationships with patients and other CUSTOMERS.

3.1 Customer Expectations: How do you listen to your patients and other customers and determine health care services to meet their needs? (40 pts.)

a. Listening to Patients and Other CUSTOMERS

(1) Current Patients and Other CUSTOMERS   HOW do you listen to, interact with, and observe patients and other CUSTOMERS to obtain actionable information? HOW do your listening methods vary for different patient groups, other CUSTOMER groups, or market SEGMENTS? HOW do your listening methods vary across the stages of patients' and other CUSTOMERS' relationships with you? HOW do you seek immediate and actionable feedback from patients and other CUSTOMERS on the quality of HEALTH CARE SERVICES, patient and other CUSTOMER support, and transactions?

(2) Potential Patients and Other CUSTOMERS   HOW do you listen to potential patients and other CUSTOMERS to obtain actionable information? HOW do you listen to former, competitors', and other potential patients and other CUSTOMERS to obtain actionable information on your HEALTH CARE SERVICES, patient and other CUSTOMER support, and transactions, as appropriate?

b. Patient and Other CUSTOMER Segmentation and Service Offerings

(1) Patient and Other CUSTOMER Segmentation   HOW do you determine your patient and other CUSTOMER groups and market SEGMENTS? HOW do you

- use information on patients, other CUSTOMERS, markets, and HEALTH CARE SERVICE offerings to identify current and anticipate future patient and other CUSTOMER groups and market SEGMENTS; and

- determine which patient and other CUSTOMER groups and market SEGMENTS to emphasize and pursue for business growth?

(2) Service Offerings   HOW do you determine HEALTH CARE SERVICE offerings? HOW do you

- determine patient, other CUSTOMER, and market needs and requirements for HEALTH CARE SERVICE offerings;

- identify and adapt HEALTH CARE SERVICE offerings to meet the requirements and exceed the expectations of your patient and other CUSTOMER groups and market SEGMENTS; and

- identify and adapt service offerings to enter new markets, to attract new patients and other CUSTOMERS, and to create opportunities to expand relationships with current patients and other CUSTOMERS, as appropriate?

Terms in SMALL CAPS are defined in the Glossary of Key Terms (pages 46–53).

Notes

3.1. Your results on performance relative to key service features should be reported in item 7.1.

3.1a(1). Your patient and other customer listening methods might include monitoring comments on social media outlets.

3.1a(1). Your listening methods should include all stages of your involvement with patients and other customers. These stages might include relationship building, the active relationship, and a follow-up strategy, as appropriate.

3.1b(2). In identifying health care service offerings, you should consider all the important characteristics of services that patients and other customers receive in each stage of their relationship with you. The focus should be on features that affect patients' and other customers' preference for and loyalty to you and your brand—for example, unique or innovative features that affect their view of clinical and service quality and that differentiate your offerings from those of competing organizations. Those latter features might include ease of access to and use of your services, including telehealth and new locations; a virtual experience; family support services; timeliness; cost; assistance with billing/administrative processes and transportation; environmental or social stewardship; and the privacy and security of patient and other customer data.

For additional guidance on this item, see the Health Care Criteria Commentary (https://www.nist.gov/baldrige /baldrige-criteria-commentary-health-care).

3.2 Customer Engagement: How do you build relationships with patients and other customers and determine satisfaction and engagement? (45 pts.)

a. Patient and Other CUSTOMER Experience

(1) Relationship Management   HOW do you build and manage relationships with patients and other CUSTOMERS? HOW do you

- acquire patients and other CUSTOMERS and build market share;
- manage and enhance your brand image;
- retain patients and other CUSTOMERS, meet their requirements, and exceed their expectations in each stage of their relationship with you?

(2) Patient and Other CUSTOMER Access and Support   HOW do you enable patients and other CUSTOMERS to seek information and support? HOW do you enable them to access your services? What are your KEY means of patient and other CUSTOMER support and communication? HOW do they vary for different patient and other CUSTOMER groups or market SEGMENTS, as appropriate? HOW do you

- determine your patients' and other CUSTOMERS' KEY support requirements, and
- DEPLOY these requirements to all people and PROCESSES involved in patient and other CUSTOMER support?

(3) Complaint Management   HOW do you manage patient and other CUSTOMER complaints? HOW do you resolve complaints promptly and effectively? HOW does your management of complaints enable you to recover your patients' and other CUSTOMERS' confidence, enhance their satisfaction and ENGAGEMENT, and avoid similar complaints in the future?

(4) Fair Treatment   How do your patient and other CUSTOMER experience PROCESSES ensure fair treatment for different patients, patient groups, other CUSTOMER groups, and market SEGMENTS?

b. Determination of Patient and Other CUSTOMER Satisfaction and ENGAGEMENT

(1) Satisfaction, Dissatisfaction, and ENGAGEMENT   HOW do you determine patient and other CUSTOMER satisfaction, dissatisfaction, and ENGAGEMENT? HOW do your determination methods differ among your patient and other CUSTOMER groups and market SEGMENTS, as appropriate? HOW do your measurements capture actionable information?

(2) Satisfaction Relative to Other Organizations   HOW do you obtain information on patients' and other CUSTOMERS' satisfaction with your organization relative to other organizations? HOW do you obtain information on your patients' and other CUSTOMERS' satisfaction

- relative to their satisfaction with your competitors; and
- relative to the satisfaction of patients and other CUSTOMERS of other organizations that provide similar HEALTH CARE SERVICES or to health care industry BENCHMARKS, as appropriate?

c. Use of VOICE-OF-THE-CUSTOMER and Market Data

HOW do you use VOICE-OF-THE-CUSTOMER and market data and information? HOW do you use VOICE-OF-THE-CUSTOMER and market data and information to build a more patient-focused culture and support operational decision making?

Terms in SMALL CAPS are defined in the Glossary of Key Terms (pages 46–53).

Notes

3.2. Results for patient and other customer perceptions and actions (outcomes) should be reported in item 7.2.

3.2a(4). You should ensure that your approaches for managing patient and other customer relationships, enabling patient and other customers to seek information and support, and managing complaints promote equity and inclusion, and that they do not inadvertently discriminate unfairly or inappropriately against specific patients or patient groups.

3.2b(1). Determining dissatisfaction should be seen as more than reviewing low satisfaction scores. It should be independently determined to identify root causes and enable a systematic remedy to avoid future dissatisfaction.

3.2b(2). Information you obtain on relative satisfaction may include comparisons with competitors; comparisons with other organizations that deliver similar health care services in a noncompetitive marketplace; or comparisons obtained through third-party surveys or surveys endorsed or required by payors, such as the Consumer Assessment of Healthcare Providers and Systems (CAHPS). Such information may also include information on why customers choose your competitors over you.

3.2c. Patient and other customer data and information should be used to support the overall performance reviews addressed in 4.1b. Voice-of-the-customer and market data and information to use might include aggregated data on complaints and, as appropriate, data and information from social media and other web-based or digital sources.

For additional guidance on this item, see the Health Care Criteria Commentary (https://www.nist.gov/baldrige /baldrige-criteria-commentary-health-care).

Measurement, Analysis, and Knowledge Management (90 pts.)

The **Measurement, ANALYSIS, and Knowledge Management** category asks HOW your organization selects, gathers, analyzes, manages, and improves its data, information, and KNOWLEDGE ASSETS; HOW it uses review findings to improve its PERFORMANCE; and HOW it learns.

4.1 Measurement, Analysis, and Improvement of Organizational Performance: **How do you measure, analyze, and then improve organizational performance?** (45 pts.)

a. **PERFORMANCE Measurement**

(1) **PERFORMANCE MEASURES   HOW do you track data and information on daily operations and overall organizational PERFORMANCE?** HOW do you

- select, collect, align, and integrate data and information to use in tracking daily operations and overall organizational PERFORMANCE; and

- track progress on achieving STRATEGIC OBJECTIVES and ACTION PLANS?

What are your KEY organizational PERFORMANCE MEASURES, including KEY short- and longer-term financial MEASURES?

(2) **Comparative Data   HOW do you select comparative data and information to support fact-based decision making?**

(3) **Measurement Agility   HOW do you ensure that your PERFORMANCE measurement system can respond to rapid or unexpected organizational or external changes, and provide timely data?**

b. **PERFORMANCE ANALYSIS and Review**

HOW do you review your organization's PERFORMANCE and capabilities? HOW do you use your KEY organizational PERFORMANCE MEASURES, as well as comparative data, in these reviews? What ANALYSES do you perform to support these reviews and ensure that conclusions are valid? HOW do your organization and its SENIOR LEADERS use these reviews to

- assess organizational success, competitive PERFORMANCE, financial health, and progress on achieving your STRATEGIC OBJECTIVES and ACTION PLANS; and

- respond rapidly to changing organizational needs and challenges in your operating environment?

HOW does your GOVERNANCE board review the organization's PERFORMANCE and its progress on STRATEGIC OBJECTIVES and ACTION PLANS, if appropriate?

c. **PERFORMANCE Improvement**

(1) **Future PERFORMANCE   HOW do you project your organization's future PERFORMANCE?** HOW do you use findings from PERFORMANCE reviews and KEY comparative and competitive data in your PROJECTIONS?

(2) **Continuous Improvement and INNOVATION   HOW do you use findings from PERFORMANCE reviews to develop priorities for continuous improvement and opportunities for INNOVATION?** HOW do you DEPLOY these priorities and opportunities

- to work group and functional-level operations; and

- when appropriate, to your suppliers, PARTNERS, and COLLABORATORS to ensure organizational ALIGNMENT?

Terms in SMALL CAPS are defined in the Glossary of Key Terms (pages 46–53).

Notes

4.1. The questions in this item are closely linked to each other and to other Health Care Criteria items. The following are examples of key linkages:

- Your organizational performance measurement (4.1a)—including the comparative data and information you select, and the performance measures you report in your Criteria item responses—should inform your organizational performance reviews (4.1b).

- Organizational performance reviews (4.1b) should reflect your strategic objectives and action plans (category 2), and the results of organizational performance analysis and review should inform your strategy development and implementation, priorities for improvement, and opportunities for innovation (4.1c).

- Your performance projections for your key action plans should be reported in 2.2a(6).

- Your organizational performance results should be reported in items 7.1–7.5.

4.1a. Data and information from performance measurement should be used to support fact-based decisions that set and align organizational directions and resource use at the work unit, key process, department, and organization levels.

4.1a(2). The comparative data and information you select should be used to support operational and strategic decision making. Comparative data and information are obtained by benchmarking and by seeking competitive comparisons. Benchmarking is identifying processes and results that represent best practices and performance for similar activities, inside or outside the health care industry. Competitive comparisons relate your performance to that of competitors and other organizations providing similar health care services.

4.1a(3). Agility in your measurement system might be necessary in response to regulatory changes, other changes in the political or societal environment, disasters and emergencies, innovations in organizational processes or business models, new competitor offerings, or productivity enhancements. Responses to such changes might involve, for example, adopting different performance measures or adjusting the intervals between measurements.

4.1b. Performance analysis includes examining performance trends; organizational, health care industry, and technology projections; and comparisons, cause-effect relationships, and correlations. This analysis should support your performance reviews, help determine root causes, and help set priorities for resource use. Accordingly, such analysis draws on all types of data: health care outcome, patient- and other customer-related, financial and market, operational, and competitive/comparative. The analysis should also draw on publicly mandated measures, when appropriate, and might also be informed by internal or external Baldrige assessments. Analysis may involve digital data analytics and data science techniques that detect patterns in large volumes of data ("big data") and interpret their meaning.

4.1b. Rapid response to changing organizational needs and challenges may include responding to the need for change in your organizational structure and work systems.

For additional guidance on this item, see the Health Care Criteria Commentary (https://www.nist.gov/baldrige /baldrige-criteria-commentary-health-care).

4.2 Information and Knowledge Management: How do you manage your information and your organizational knowledge assets? (45 pts.)

a. Data and Information

(1) Quality   HOW do you verify and ensure the quality of organizational data and information? HOW do you manage digital and other data and information to ensure their accuracy and validity, integrity and reliability, and currency?

(2) Availability   HOW do you ensure the availability of organizational data and information? HOW do you make needed data and information available in a user-friendly format and timely manner to your WORKFORCE, suppliers, PARTNERS, COLLABORATORS, patients, and other CUSTOMERS, as appropriate? HOW do you ensure that your information technology systems are reliable and user-friendly?

b. Organizational Knowledge

(1) Knowledge Management   HOW do you build and manage organizational knowledge? HOW do you

- collect and transfer WORKFORCE knowledge;
- blend and correlate data from different sources to build new knowledge;
- transfer relevant knowledge from and to patients, other CUSTOMERS, suppliers, PARTNERS, and COLLABORATORS; and
- assemble and transfer relevant knowledge for use in your INNOVATION and strategic planning PROCESSES?

(2) Best Practices   HOW do you share best practices in your organization? HOW do you identify internal and external organizational units or operations that are HIGH PERFORMING? HOW do you identify best practices for sharing and implement them across your organization, as appropriate?

(3) Organizational LEARNING   HOW do you use your knowledge and resources to embed LEARNING in the way your organization operates?

Terms in SMALL CAPS are defined in the Glossary of Key Terms (pages 46–53).

Notes

4.2a(2). Information technology systems include, for example, physical devices and systems; software platforms and applications; and externally based or shared information systems, such as those stored in the cloud or outside your organization's control. Your response might include information related to the interoperability and effective use of electronic health records within your organization.

4.2a(2). The security and cybersecurity of your information technology systems are addressed as part of your overall security and cybersecurity system in item 6.2. That system involves managing and reducing risks to operational systems as well as to data and information.

4.2b(1). Building and managing organizational knowledge from different sources may involve handling big data sets and disparate types of structured and unstructured data and information, such as data tables, video, audio, photos,

and text. Blending and correlating data may involve using artificial intelligence, digital data analytics, and data science techniques that detect patterns in large volumes of data and interpret their meaning. Using these techniques to make decisions with human consequences requires deploying technology and leveraging data in a way that protects information about organizations and individuals.

4.2b(3). Embedding learning in the way your organization operates means that learning (1) is a part of everyday work; (2) results in solving problems at their source; (3) is focused on building and sharing knowledge throughout your organization; and (4) is driven by opportunities to bring about significant, meaningful change and to innovate.

For additional guidance on this item, see the Health Care Criteria Commentary (https://www.nist.gov/baldrige /baldrige-criteria-commentary-health-care).

5 Workforce (85 pts.)

The **WORKFORCE** category asks HOW your organization assesses WORKFORCE CAPABILITY and CAPACITY needs and builds a WORKFORCE environment that is conducive to HIGH PERFORMANCE. The category also asks HOW your organization engages, manages, and develops your WORKFORCE to utilize its full potential in alignment with your organization's overall needs.

5.1 Workforce Environment: How do you build an effective and supportive workforce environment? (40 pts.)

a. WORKFORCE CAPABILITY and CAPACITY

(1) **CAPABILITY and CAPACITY Needs**   **HOW do you assess your WORKFORCE CAPABILITY and CAPACITY needs?** HOW do you assess the skills, competencies, certifications, and staffing levels you need in the short and long term?

(2) **New WORKFORCE Members**   **HOW do you recruit, hire, and onboard new WORKFORCE members?** HOW do you ensure that your WORKFORCE represents the DIVERSITY of ideas, cultures, and thinking in your hiring and patient communities? HOW do you ensure the fit of new WORKFORCE members with your organizational culture?

(3) **WORKFORCE Change**   **HOW do you prepare your WORKFORCE for changing CAPABILITY and CAPACITY needs?** HOW do you

- balance the needs of your WORKFORCE and your organization to ensure continuity, prevent WORKFORCE reductions, and minimize the impact of any necessary reductions;
- prepare for and manage any periods of WORKFORCE growth; and
- prepare your WORKFORCE for changes in organizational structure, workplaces, WORK SYSTEMS, and technology when needed?

(4) **Work Accomplishment**   **HOW do you organize and manage your WORKFORCE?** HOW do you organize and manage your WORKFORCE to

- capitalize on your organization's CORE COMPETENCIES;
- reinforce organizational RESILIENCE, agility, and a patient/other CUSTOMER and business focus; and
- exceed PERFORMANCE expectations?

b. Workplace Climate

(1) **Workplace Environment**   **HOW do you ensure workplace health, security, and accessibility for the WORKFORCE?** What are your PERFORMANCE MEASURES and improvement GOALS for your workplace environmental factors?

(2) **WORKFORCE Benefits and Policies**   **HOW do you support your WORKFORCE via services, benefits, and policies?** HOW do you tailor these to the needs of a diverse WORKFORCE and different WORKFORCE groups and SEGMENTS?

Terms in SMALL CAPS are defined in the Glossary of Key Terms (pages 46–53).

Notes

5. Results related to workforce environment and engagement should be reported in item 7.3. People supervised by a contractor should be addressed in categories 2 and 6 as part of your larger work system strategy and your internal work processes. For organizations that also rely on volunteers, the workforce includes these volunteers. Workforce approaches should include these volunteers as appropriate to the functions they fulfill for the organization.

5.1a(1). Your assessment of workforce capability and capacity needs should consider not only current needs, but also future requirements based on the strategic objectives and action plans you identify in category 2 and the future performance you discuss in 4.1c(1).

5.1a(3). Preparing your workforce for change might include preparing for alternate workplaces or telework, or for changes in patient, other customer, or service requirements that lead to the use of new technology or redesigned work systems. Such preparation might include training, education, frequent communication, consideration of workforce employment and employability, career counseling, and outplacement and other services.

5.1a(3), 5.1a(4). The way you organize and manage your workforce may be influenced by changes in your internal or external environment, culture, or strategic objectives.

5.1b(1). Workplace accessibility maximizes productivity by eliminating barriers that can prevent people with disabilities from working to their potential. A fully inclusive workplace is physically, technologically, and attitudinally accessible without bias.

5.1b(1). If workplace environmental factors and their performance measures or targets differ significantly for your different workplace environments, you should include these differences in your response. You should address workplace safety in item 6.2 as part of your overall safety system, which also ensures the safety of all other people in your workplace.

For additional guidance on this item, see the Health Care Criteria Commentary (https://www.nist.gov/baldrige/baldrige-criteria-commentary-health-care).

5.2 Workforce Engagement: How do you engage your workforce for retention and high performance? (45 pts.)

PROCESS

a. Assessment of WORKFORCE ENGAGEMENT

    (1) **Drivers of ENGAGEMENT   HOW do you determine the KEY drivers of WORKFORCE ENGAGEMENT?** HOW do you determine these drivers for different WORKFORCE groups and SEGMENTS?

    (2) **Assessment of ENGAGEMENT   HOW do you assess WORKFORCE ENGAGEMENT?** What formal and informal assessment methods and MEASURES do you use to determine WORKFORCE satisfaction and WORKFORCE ENGAGEMENT? HOW do these methods and MEASURES differ across WORKFORCE groups and SEGMENTS? HOW do you also use other INDICATORS to assess and improve WORKFORCE ENGAGEMENT?

b. Organizational Culture

HOW do you foster an organizational culture that is characterized by open communication, HIGH PERFORMANCE, patient safety, and an engaged WORKFORCE? HOW do you reinforce your organizational culture? HOW do you ensure that your organizational culture supports your VISION and VALUES; promotes equity and inclusion; and benefits from the DIVERSITY of the ideas, cultures, and thinking in your WORKFORCE? HOW do you EMPOWER your WORKFORCE?

c. PERFORMANCE Management and Development

    (1) **PERFORMANCE Management   HOW does your WORKFORCE PERFORMANCE management system support HIGH PERFORMANCE?** HOW does it consider WORKFORCE compensation, reward, recognition, and incentive practices? HOW does it reinforce INTELLIGENT RISK taking, a patient/other CUSTOMER and business focus, and achievement of your ACTION PLANS?

    (2) **PERFORMANCE Development   HOW does your LEARNING and development system support the personal development of WORKFORCE members and your organization's needs?** HOW does it consider the LEARNING and development desires of WORKFORCE members, support organizational PERFORMANCE improvement and INTELLIGENT RISK taking, and support ethical health care and ethical business practices?

    (3) **LEARNING and Development EFFECTIVENESS   HOW do you evaluate the EFFECTIVENESS of your LEARNING and development system?** HOW do you

        • correlate LEARNING and development outcomes with findings from your assessment of WORKFORCE ENGAGEMENT and with KEY organizational RESULTS, and

        • use these correlations to identify opportunities for improvement both in WORKFORCE ENGAGEMENT and in LEARNING and development offerings?

    (4) **Career Development   HOW do you manage career development for your WORKFORCE and your future leaders?** HOW do you carry out succession planning for management, leadership, and other KEY positions?

    (5) **Equity and Inclusion   HOW do you ensure that your performance management, performance development, and career development approaches promote equity and inclusion for a diverse WORKFORCE and different WORKFORCE groups and SEGMENTS?**

Terms in SMALL CAPS are defined in the Glossary of Key Terms (pages 46–53).

Notes

5.2a(1). Drivers of workforce engagement (identified in P.1a[3]) refer to the drivers of workforce members' commitment, both emotional and intellectual, to accomplishing the organization's work, mission, and vision.

5.2a(2). Other indicators to use in assessing and improving workforce engagement might include workforce retention, absenteeism, grievances, safety, and productivity.

5.2c(2). Your response should include how you address any considerations for workforce development, learning, and career progression that are unique to your organization. These might include development opportunities that address your organization's core competencies, strategic challenges, and action plans, including those related to high reliability; organizational change and innovation; improvements in delivering a positive patient and other customer experience; and the reinforcement of new knowledge and skills on the job. Your response should also consider the breadth of development opportunities you might offer, including education, training, coaching, mentoring, and work-related experiences.

For additional guidance on this item, see the Health Care Criteria Commentary (https://www.nist.gov/baldrige /baldrige-criteria-commentary-health-care).

6 Operations (85 pts.)

The **Operations** category asks HOW your organization designs, manages, improves, and innovates its HEALTH CARE SERVICES and WORK PROCESSES and improves operational effectiveness to deliver VALUE to patients and other CUSTOMERS and to achieve ongoing organizational success.

6.1 Work Processes: How do you design, manage, and improve your key health care services and work processes? (45 pts.)

a. Service and PROCESS Design

(1) **Determination of Service and PROCESS Requirements** **HOW do you determine** KEY HEALTH CARE SERVICE and **WORK PROCESS requirements?**

(2) **KEY WORK PROCESSES** **What are your organization's** KEY WORK PROCESSES? What are the KEY requirements for these WORK PROCESSES?

(3) **Design Concepts** **HOW do you design your** HEALTH CARE SERVICES **and** WORK PROCESSES **to meet requirements?** HOW do you incorporate new technology, organizational knowledge, evidence-based medicine, HEALTH CARE SERVICE excellence, patient and other CUSTOMER VALUE, consideration of risk, and the potential need for agility into these services and PROCESSES?

b. PROCESS Management and Improvement

(1) **PROCESS Implementation** **HOW does your day-to-day operation of** WORK PROCESSES **ensure that they meet KEY PROCESS requirements?** What KEY PERFORMANCE MEASURES or INDICATORS and in-process MEASURES do you use to control and improve your WORK PROCESSES? HOW do these MEASURES relate to the quality of outcomes and MEASURES of the PERFORMANCE of your HEALTH CARE SERVICES?

(2) **Patient Expectations and Preferences** **HOW do you address and consider each patient's expectations?** HOW do you explain HEALTH CARE SERVICE delivery PROCESSES and likely outcomes to set realistic patient expectations? HOW do you factor patient decision making and patient preferences into the delivery of HEALTH CARE SERVICES?

(3) **Support PROCESSES** **HOW do you determine your** KEY support PROCESSES? What are your KEY support PROCESSES? HOW does your day-to-day operation of these PROCESSES ensure that they meet KEY organizational requirements?

(4) **Service and PROCESS Improvement** **HOW do you improve your** WORK PROCESSES **and support** PROCESSES **to improve** HEALTH CARE SERVICES **and** PERFORMANCE, **enhance your** CORE COMPETENCIES, **and reduce variability?**

c. Supply-Network Management

HOW do you manage your supply network? HOW do you select suppliers that are qualified and positioned to meet your operational needs, enhance your PERFORMANCE, support your STRATEGIC OBJECTIVES, and enhance your patients' and other CUSTOMERS' satisfaction? HOW do you

- promote ALIGNMENT and collaboration within your supply network;
- ensure supply-network agility and RESILIENCE in responding to changes in patient, other CUSTOMER, market, and organizational requirements; and
- communicate PERFORMANCE expectations, measure and evaluate suppliers' PERFORMANCE, provide feedback to help them improve, and deal with poorly performing suppliers?

d. Management of Opportunities for INNOVATION

HOW do you pursue your identified opportunities for INNOVATION? HOW do you pursue the STRATEGIC OPPORTUNITIES that you have determined are INTELLIGENT RISKS? HOW do you make financial and other resources available to pursue these opportunities? HOW do you decide to discontinue pursuing them at the appropriate time?

Terms in SMALL CAPS are defined in the Glossary of Key Terms (pages 46–53).

Notes

6.1. The results of improvements in the performance of your health care services and processes should be reported in item 7.1.

6.1a(3). Process design also includes the need to extensively redesign a process due to changes in requirements or technology, or the need to incorporate digital technology, such as enhanced automation, the Internet of Things, artificial intelligence, and cloud operations. Agility may be needed when work processes need to change as a result of overall work system changes, such as bringing a supply-network product, service, or process in-house to avoid disruptions in supply due to unpredictable external events, or outsourcing a product, service, or process formerly carried out in-house.

6.1b(3). Your key support processes should support your value-creation processes. They might include processes that support leaders and other workforce members engaged in, for example, service design and delivery, patient and other customer interactions, and business and enterprise management. Examples might include accounting and purchasing.

6.1b(4). Your approaches to improve process performance and reduce variability should be part of the performance improvement system you describe in P.2c in the Organizational Profile.

6.1c. To ensure that suppliers are positioned to meet operational needs and enhance your performance and your patients' and other customers' satisfaction, you might partner with suppliers or form alliances among multiple organizations within the supply network for mutual benefit. Communication of expectations and feedback to suppliers should be two-way, allowing suppliers to express what they need from you and other organizations within the supply network. For many organizations, these mechanisms may change as marketplace, patient, other customer, or stakeholder requirements change.

6.1d. Your process for pursuing opportunities for innovation should capitalize on strategic opportunities identified as intelligent risks in 2.1a(2). It should also include other intelligent risks, such as those arising from your performance reviews (4.1c[2]), your knowledge management approaches (4.2b), and other sources of potential innovations.

For additional guidance on this item, see the Health Care Criteria Commentary (https://www.nist.gov/baldrige /baldrige-criteria-commentary-health-care).

6.2 Operational Effectiveness: **How do you ensure effective management of your operations?** (40 pts.)

a. PROCESS Efficiency and EFFECTIVENESS

HOW do you manage the cost, efficiency, and EFFECTIVENESS of your operations? HOW do you

- incorporate cycle time, PRODUCTIVITY, and other efficiency and EFFECTIVENESS factors into your WORK PROCESSES;
- prevent rework and errors;
- minimize the costs of inspections, tests, and PROCESS or PERFORMANCE audits, as appropriate; and
- balance the need for cost control and efficiency with the needs of your patients and other CUSTOMERS?

b. Security and Cybersecurity

HOW do you ensure the security and cybersecurity of sensitive or privileged data and information and of KEY assets? HOW do you manage physical and digital data, information, and KEY operational systems to ensure confidentiality and only appropriate physical and digital access? HOW do you

- maintain your awareness of emerging security and cybersecurity threats;
- ensure that your WORKFORCE, patients, other CUSTOMERS, PARTNERS, and suppliers understand and fulfill their security and cybersecurity roles and responsibilities;
- identify and prioritize KEY information technology and operational systems to secure; and
- protect these systems from potential cybersecurity events, detect cybersecurity events, and respond to and recover from cybersecurity incidents?

c. Safety, Business Continuity, and RESILIENCE

(1) Safety **HOW do you provide a safe operating environment for your WORKFORCE and other people in your workplace?** HOW does your safety system address prevention, inspection, root-cause ANALYSIS of failures, and recovery?

(2) Patient Safety **HOW do you reduce patient harm and medical errors?** HOW does your patient safety system address prevention, root-cause ANALYSIS of failures, and recovery?

(3) Business Continuity and RESILIENCE **HOW do you ensure that your organization can anticipate, prepare for, and recover from disasters, emergencies, and other disruptions?** HOW do you consider risk, prevention, protection, continuity of operations, and recovery in the event of disruptions? HOW do you take into account patient, other CUSTOMER, and business needs, and your reliance on your WORKFORCE, supply network, PARTNERS, and information technology systems?

Terms in SMALL CAPS are defined in the Glossary of Key Terms (pages 46–53).

Notes

6.2b. For examples of what your information technology systems might include, see the note to 4.2a(2).

6.2b. Managing cybersecurity includes protecting against the loss of sensitive information about employees, patients, other customers, and organizations; protecting assets, including intellectual property; and protecting against the financial, legal, and reputational aspects of breaches. Many sources for general and industry-specific cybersecurity standards and practices are referenced in the *Framework for Improving Critical Infrastructure Cybersecurity* (https://www.nist.gov/cyberframework). The *Baldrige Cybersecurity Excellence Builder* (https://www.nist.gov/baldrige/products-services) is a self-assessment tool incorporating the concepts of the Cybersecurity Framework and the Baldrige systems perspective.

6.2c(3). Disasters and emergencies might be short- or longer-term and might be related to weather, climate, utilities, security, or a local or national health or other emergency. The extent to which you prepare for such events will depend on your organization's environment and its sensitivity to short- or longer-term disruptions of operations. Acceptable levels of risk will vary depending on the nature of your health care services, supply network, and stakeholder needs and expectations.

For additional guidance on this item, see the Health Care Criteria Commentary (https://www.nist.gov/baldrige /baldrige-criteria-commentary-health-care).

7 Results (450 pts.)

The **RESULTS** category asks about your organization's PERFORMANCE and improvement in all KEY areas—health care and PROCESS RESULTS; CUSTOMER RESULTS; WORKFORCE RESULTS; leadership and GOVERNANCE RESULTS; and financial, market, and strategy RESULTS.

7.1 Health Care and Process Results: What are your health care and process effectiveness results? (120 pts.)

a. Health Care and CUSTOMER-Focused Service RESULTS

What are your health care RESULTS and your RESULTS for your patient and other CUSTOMER service processes? What are your RESULTS for KEY MEASURES or INDICATORS of health care outcomes and the PERFORMANCE of services that are important to and directly serve your patients and other CUSTOMERS? HOW do these RESULTS differ by HEALTH CARE SERVICE offerings, patient and other CUSTOMER groups, and market SEGMENTS, as appropriate?

b. WORK PROCESS EFFECTIVENESS RESULTS

(1) PROCESS EFFECTIVENESS and Efficiency **What are your PROCESS EFFECTIVENESS and efficiency RESULTS?** What are your RESULTS for KEY MEASURES or INDICATORS of the operational PERFORMANCE of your KEY work and support PROCESSES, including PRODUCTIVITY, cycle time, patient safety, and other appropriate MEASURES of PROCESS EFFECTIVENESS, efficiency, security and cybersecurity, and INNOVATION? How do these RESULTS differ by PROCESS types, as appropriate?

(2) Safety and Emergency Preparedness **What are your safety and emergency preparedness RESULTS?** What are your RESULTS for KEY MEASURES or INDICATORS of the EFFECTIVENESS of your organization's safety system and its preparedness for disasters or emergencies? How do these RESULTS differ by location or PROCESS type, as appropriate?

c. Supply-Network Management RESULTS

What are your supply-network management RESULTS? What are your RESULTS for KEY MEASURES or INDICATORS of the PERFORMANCE of your supply network, including its contribution to enhancing your PERFORMANCE?

Terms in SMALL CAPS are defined in the Glossary of Key Terms (pages 46–53).

Notes

7. There is not a one-to-one correspondence between results items and Criteria categories 1–6. Results should be considered systemically, with contributions to individual results items frequently stemming from processes in more than one Criteria category.

The Baldrige scoring system (pages 29–34) asks for current, trended, comparative, and segmented data, as appropriate, to provide key information for analyzing and reviewing your organizational performance (item 4.1), to demonstrate use of organizational knowledge (item 4.2), and to provide the operational basis for patient- and other customer-focused results (item 7.2) and financial, market, and strategy results (item 7.5).

In a few areas, your results may be qualitative or not amenable to trending over time. Some examples are results for governance accountability, training hours for suppliers on new services or processes, and results for limited or one-time projects or processes.

Comparative data and information are obtained by benchmarking (inside and outside your industry, as appropriate) and by seeking competitive comparisons. In a few cases,

such as results for projects or processes that are unique to your organization, comparative data may not be available or appropriate.

7.1. Results should include those for representative key measures that are publicly reported and/or mandated by regulators, accreditors, or payors, such as the Healthcare Effectiveness Data and Information Set (HEDIS); Centers for Medicare and Medicaid Services (CMS) measures, including outpatient measures; and Agency for Healthcare Research and Quality (AHRQ) measures, as appropriate.

7.1a. Health care results and results for patient and other customer service processes should relate to the key requirements and expectations you identify in P.1b(2), which are based on information gathered through processes you describe in category 3. The measures or indicators should address factors that affect patient and other customer preference, such as those listed in the notes to P.1b(2) and 3.1b.

7.1b. Results should address the key operational requirements you identify in the Organizational Profile and in category 6.

7.1b. Appropriate measures and indicators of work process effectiveness might include medical error rates; rate of and reduction in serious safety events; timeliness of care delivery; results for externally provided health care services and processes; rates and results of health care service and work system innovation; work layout improvements; changes in supervisory ratios; Occupational Safety and Health Administration (OSHA)-reportable incidents; measures or indicators of the success of emergency drills or simulations, such as cycle time, containment, and the meeting of standards; and results for work relocation or contingency exercises.

7.1c. Appropriate measures and indicators of supply-network performance might include supplier and partner audits; just-in-time delivery; and acceptance results for externally provided services and processes. Measures and indicators of contributions to enhancing your performance might include those for improvements in downstream supplier services delivered directly to patients and other customers.

For additional guidance on this item, see the Health Care Criteria Commentary (https://www.nist.gov/baldrige /baldrige-criteria-commentary-health-care).

7.2 Customer Results: **What are your customer-focused performance results? (80 pts.)**

a. Patient- and Other CUSTOMER-Focused RESULTS

(1) **Patient and Other CUSTOMER Satisfaction** **What are your patient and other CUSTOMER satisfaction and dissatisfaction RESULTS?** What are your RESULTS for KEY MEASURES or INDICATORS of patient and other CUSTOMER satisfaction and dissatisfaction? How do these RESULTS differ by HEALTH CARE SERVICE offerings, patient and other CUSTOMER groups, and market SEGMENTS, as appropriate?

(2) **Patient and Other CUSTOMER ENGAGEMENT** **What are your patient and other CUSTOMER ENGAGEMENT RESULTS?** What are your RESULTS for KEY MEASURES or INDICATORS of patient and other CUSTOMER ENGAGEMENT, including those for building relationships with patients and other CUSTOMERS? How do these RESULTS compare over the course of your patients' and other CUSTOMERS' relationships with you, as appropriate? How do these RESULTS differ by HEALTH CARE SERVICE offerings, patient and other CUSTOMER groups, and market SEGMENTS, as appropriate?

Terms in SMALL CAPS are defined in the Glossary of Key Terms (pages 46–53).

RESULTS

Notes

7.2. Results for patient and other customer satisfaction, dissatisfaction, and engagement should relate to the patient and other customer groups and market segments you identify in P.1b(2) and to the listening and determination methods you report in category 3.

7.2a(1). Results from any of the CAHPS surveys should be included if your organization reports these measures.

For additional guidance on this item, see the Health Care Criteria Commentary (https://www.nist.gov/baldrige /baldrige-criteria-commentary-health-care).

7.3 Workforce Results: What are your workforce-focused performance results? (80 pts.)

a. WORKFORCE-Focused RESULTS

(1) WORKFORCE CAPABILITY and CAPACITY **What are your WORKFORCE CAPABILITY and CAPACITY RESULTS?** What are your RESULTS for KEY MEASURES of WORKFORCE CAPABILITY and CAPACITY, including appropriate skills and staffing levels? How do these RESULTS differ by the DIVERSITY of your WORKFORCE and by your WORKFORCE groups and SEGMENTS, as appropriate?

(2) Workplace Climate **What are your workplace climate RESULTS?** What are your RESULTS for KEY MEASURES or INDICATORS of your workplace climate, including those for WORKFORCE health, security, accessibility, and services and benefits, as appropriate? How do these RESULTS differ by the DIVERSITY of your WORKFORCE and by your WORKFORCE groups and SEGMENTS, as appropriate?

(3) WORKFORCE ENGAGEMENT **What are your WORKFORCE ENGAGEMENT RESULTS?** What are your RESULTS for KEY MEASURES or INDICATORS of WORKFORCE satisfaction and WORKFORCE ENGAGEMENT? How do these RESULTS differ by the DIVERSITY of your WORKFORCE and by your WORKFORCE groups and SEGMENTS, as appropriate?

(4) WORKFORCE Development **What are your WORKFORCE and leader development RESULTS?** What are your RESULTS for KEY MEASURES or INDICATORS of WORKFORCE and leader development? How do these RESULTS differ by the DIVERSITY of your WORKFORCE and by your WORKFORCE groups and SEGMENTS, as appropriate?

Terms in SMALL CAPS are defined in the Glossary of Key Terms (pages 46–53).

Note

7.3. Results reported in this item should relate to the processes, measures, and indicators you report in category 5. Your results should also respond to the key work process needs you report in category 6 and to the action plans and workforce plans you report in item 2.2. Responses should include results for independent practitioners, volunteers, and health profession students, as appropriate.

For additional guidance on this item, see the Health Care Criteria Commentary (https://www.nist.gov/baldrige /baldrige-criteria-commentary-health-care).

7.4 Leadership and Governance Results: What are your senior leadership and governance results? (80 pts.)

a. Leadership, GOVERNANCE, and Societal Contribution RESULTS

(1) Leadership **What are your RESULTS for SENIOR LEADERS' communication and engagement with the WORKFORCE, PARTNERS, patients, and other CUSTOMERS?** What are your RESULTS for KEY MEASURES or INDICATORS of SENIOR LEADERS' communication and engagement with the WORKFORCE, PARTNERS, patients, and other CUSTOMERS to DEPLOY your VISION and VALUES, encourage two-way communication, cultivate INNOVATION and INTELLIGENT RISK taking, and create a focus on action? How do these RESULTS differ by organizational units and by patient and other CUSTOMER groups, as appropriate?

(2) GOVERNANCE **What are your RESULTS for GOVERNANCE accountability?** What are your RESULTS for KEY MEASURES or INDICATORS of GOVERNANCE and internal and external fiscal accountability, as appropriate?

(3) Law, Regulation, and Accreditation **What are your legal, regulatory, and accreditation RESULTS?** What are your RESULTS for KEY MEASURES or INDICATORS of meeting and surpassing regulatory, legal, and accreditation requirements? How do these RESULTS differ by organizational units, as appropriate?

(4) Ethics **What are your RESULTS for ETHICAL BEHAVIOR?** What are your RESULTS for KEY MEASURES or INDICATORS of ETHICAL BEHAVIOR, breaches of ETHICAL BEHAVIOR, and STAKEHOLDER trust in your SENIOR LEADERS and GOVERNANCE? How do these RESULTS differ by organizational units, as appropriate?

(5) Society **What are your RESULTS for societal well-being and support of your KEY communities?** What are your RESULTS for KEY MEASURES or INDICATORS of your societal contributions, support of your KEY communities, and contributions to community health?

Terms in SMALL CAPS are defined in the Glossary of Key Terms (pages 46–53).

(Item notes are on the next page.)

Notes

7.4. Responses should relate to the communication processes you identify in item 1.1 and the governance, legal and regulatory, ethics, and societal contribution processes and measures you report in item 1.2. Workforce-related occupational safety and health results (e.g., OSHA-reportable incidents) should be reported in 7.1b(2) and 7.3a(2).

7.4a(2). Responses might include financial statement issues and risks, important internal and external auditor recommendations, and management's responses to these matters.

7.4a(4). For examples of measures of ethical behavior and stakeholder trust, see the note to 1.2b(2).

7.4a(5). Measures of contributions to societal well-being might include those for reduced energy consumption, the use of renewable energy resources and recycled water, reduction of your carbon footprint, waste reduction and utilization, and alternative approaches to conserving resources (e.g., increased virtual meetings).

For additional guidance on this item, see the Health Care Criteria Commentary (https://www.nist.gov/baldrige /baldrige-criteria-commentary-health-care).

7.5 Financial, Market, and Strategy Results: What are your results for financial viability and strategy implementation? (90 pts.)

a. Financial and Market RESULTS

(1) Financial PERFORMANCE **What are your financial PERFORMANCE RESULTS?** What are your RESULTS for KEY MEASURES or INDICATORS of financial PERFORMANCE, including aggregate MEASURES of financial return, financial viability, and budgetary PERFORMANCE, as appropriate? How do these RESULTS differ by market SEGMENTS and patient and other CUSTOMER groups, as appropriate?

(2) Marketplace PERFORMANCE **What are your marketplace PERFORMANCE RESULTS?** What are your RESULTS for KEY MEASURES or INDICATORS of marketplace PERFORMANCE, including market share or position, market and market share growth, and new markets entered, as appropriate? How do these RESULTS differ by market SEGMENTS and patient and other CUSTOMER groups, as appropriate?

b. Strategy Implementation RESULTS

What are your RESULTS for achievement of your organizational strategy and ACTION PLANS? What are your RESULTS for KEY MEASURES or INDICATORS of achievement of your organizational strategy and ACTION PLANS? What are your RESULTS for taking INTELLIGENT RISKS?

RESULTS

Terms in SMALL CAPS are defined in the Glossary of Key Terms (pages 46–53).

Notes

7.5a. Results should relate to the financial measures you report in 4.1a(1) and the financial management approaches you report in item 2.2.

7.5a(1). Aggregate measures of financial return might include those for return on investment (ROI), operating margins, profitability, or profitability by key heath care service. Measures of financial viability might include those for liquidity, debt-to-equity ratio, days cash on hand, asset utilization, cash flow, bond ratings, accountable care organization or shared savings programs, and value-based purchasing financial results, as appropriate. For nonprofit health care organizations, measures of performance to budget might include additions to or subtractions from reserve funds, cost avoidance or savings, responses to

budget decreases, lowering of costs to patients or other customers or return of funds as a result of increased efficiency, administrative expenditures as a percentage of budget, and the cost of fundraising versus funds raised.

7.5b. Measures or indicators of strategy and action plan achievement should relate to the strategic objectives and goals you report in 2.1b(1), the elements of risk you report in 2.1a(3), and the action plan performance measures and projected performance you report in 2.2a(5) and 2.2a(6), respectively.

For additional guidance on this item, see the Health Care Criteria Commentary (https://www.nist.gov/baldrige /baldrige-criteria-commentary-health-care).

Scoring System

The scoring of responses to Health Care Criteria for Performance Excellence items is based on two evaluation dimensions: process (categories 1–6) and results (category 7).

To score Health Care Criteria responses, consider the following information relative to the item questions and the scoring guidelines (pages 32–33):

- The key organization factors presented in the Organizational Profile

- The maturity and appropriateness of the approaches, the breadth of their deployment, and the strengths of the learning and improvement process

- The level of performance and how results compare to those of other, relevant organizations or benchmarks

Scoring Dimensions

Process

Process refers to the methods your organization uses and improves. Processes address the questions in categories 1–6. The four factors used to evaluate process are *approach, deployment, learning,* and *integration* (ADLI). Baldrige-based feedback reflects strengths and opportunities for improvement in these factors. A score for a process item is based on a holistic assessment of your overall performance, taking into account the four process factors.

Approach comprises

- the methods used to carry out the process,

- the appropriateness of these methods to the item questions and your operating environment,

- the effectiveness of your use of the methods, and

- the degree to which the approach is repeatable and based on reliable data and information (i.e., systematic).

Deployment is the extent to which

- your approach addresses item questions that are relevant and important to your organization,

- your approach is applied consistently, and

- your approach is used by all appropriate work units.

Learning comprises

- the refinement of your approach through cycles of evaluation and improvement,

- the adoption of best practices or innovations to improve your approach, and

- the sharing of refinements and innovations with other relevant work units and processes in your organization.

See "From Fighting Fires to Innovation" on page 34, which illustrates a progression through the maturity levels for this scoring dimension.

Integration is the extent to which

- your approach is aligned with the organizational needs identified in the Organizational Profile and other process items;

- your measures, information, and improvement systems are complementary across processes and work units; and

- your plans, processes, results, analyses, learning, and actions are harmonized across processes and work units to support organization-wide goals.

In scoring process items, keep in mind that approach, deployment, learning, and integration are linked. Descriptions of approach should always indicate the deployment—consistent with the specific questions in the item and your organization. As processes mature, the description should also show cycles of learning (including innovation), as well as integration with other processes and work units (see "Steps toward Mature Processes," page 31).

Results

Results are the outputs and outcomes your organization achieves, which address the questions in category 7. The four factors used to evaluate results are *levels, trends, comparisons,* and *integration* (LeTCI). A score for a results item is based on a holistic assessment of your overall performance, taking into account the four results factors.

Levels are your current performance on a meaningful measurement scale.

Trends comprise your rate of performance improvement or continuation of good performance in areas of importance (i.e., the slope of data points over time).

Comparisons comprise your performance relative to that of other, appropriate organizations, such as competitors or organizations similar to yours, or benchmarks.

Integration is the extent to which your results measures (often through segmentation) address important performance requirements relating to patients, other customers, health care services, markets, processes, action plans, and organization-wide goals identified in your Organizational Profile and in process items.

In the scoring of results items, look for data on performance levels, trends, and relevant comparisons for key measures and indicators of your organization's performance, as well as integration with your organization's key requirements. Results items should also show data on the breadth of the performance results reported. This is directly related to deployment and organizational learning; if improvement processes are widely shared and deployed, there should be corresponding results.

"Importance" as a Scoring Consideration

A critical consideration in Baldrige evaluation and feedback is the importance of your reported processes and results to your key business factors. The areas of greatest importance should be identified in your Organizational Profile and in items such as 2.1, 2.2, 3.2, 5.1, 5.2, and 6.1. Your key patient and other customer requirements, competitive environment, workforce needs, key strategic objectives, and action plans are particularly important.

How to Score an Item Response

Follow these steps in assigning a score to an item response.

Read the scoring guidelines (pages 32–33).

Choose the scoring range (e.g., 30–45%, 50–65%, or 70–85%) that is most descriptive of the organization's achievement level as presented in the item response.

Choose this range based on a holistic view of either the four process factors (ADLI) or the four results factors (LeTCI) in aggregate. In this holistic view, the scoring range to assign is the one that best reflects the applicant's response as a whole; do not tally or average independent assessments of each of the four factors. No one evaluation factor serves as a "gate" that keeps the score out of a higher range.

The "most descriptive" range is not necessarily a perfect fit. It often reflects some gaps between the response and the description of one or more of the factors in the chosen scoring range.

Read the next higher and the next lower scoring ranges. Assign a score (e.g., 75% or 80%) within the chosen range by evaluating whether the item response as a whole is closer to the statements in the next higher or the next lower scoring range.

Steps toward Mature Processes

An Aid for Assessing and Scoring Process Items

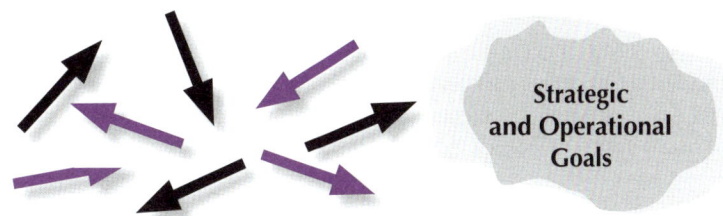

Reacting to Problems (0–25%)

Operations are characterized by activities rather than by processes, and they are largely responsive to immediate needs or problems. Goals are poorly defined.

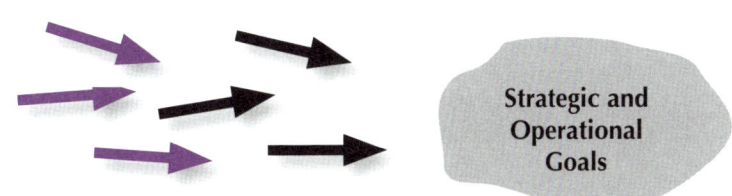

Early Systematic Approaches (30–45%)

The organization is beginning to carry out operations with repeatable processes, evaluation, and improvement, and there is some early coordination among organizational units. Strategy and quantitative goals are being defined.

Aligned Approaches (50–65%)

Operations are characterized by repeatable processes that are regularly evaluated for improvement. Learnings are shared, and there is coordination among organizational units. Processes address key strategies and goals.

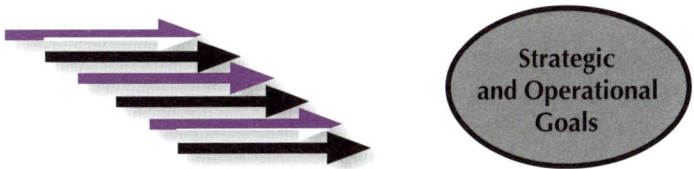

Integrated Approaches (70–100%)

Operations are characterized by repeatable processes that are regularly evaluated for change and improvement in collaboration with other affected units. The organization seeks and achieves efficiencies across units through analysis, innovation, and the sharing of information and knowledge. Processes and measures track progress on key strategic and operational goals.

Process Scoring Guidelines (For Use with Categories 1–6)

SCORE	DESCRIPTION
0% or 5%	• No SYSTEMATIC APPROACH to item questions is evident; information is ANECDOTAL. (A) • Little or no DEPLOYMENT of any SYSTEMATIC APPROACH is evident. (D) • An improvement orientation is not evident; improvement is achieved by reacting to problems. (L) • No organizational ALIGNMENT is evident; individual areas or work units operate independently. (I)
10%, 15%, 20%, or 25%	• The beginning of a SYSTEMATIC APPROACH to the BASIC QUESTION in the item is evident. (A) • The APPROACH is in the early stages of DEPLOYMENT in most areas or work units, inhibiting progress in achieving the BASIC QUESTION in the item. (D) • Early stages of a transition from reacting to problems to a general improvement orientation are evident. (L) • The APPROACH is ALIGNED with other areas or work units largely through joint problem solving. (I)
30%, 35%, 40%, or 45%	• An EFFECTIVE, SYSTEMATIC APPROACH, responsive to the BASIC QUESTION in the item, is evident. (A) • The APPROACH is DEPLOYED, although some areas or work units are in early stages of DEPLOYMENT. (D) • The beginning of a SYSTEMATIC APPROACH to evaluation and improvement of KEY PROCESSES is evident. (L) • The APPROACH is in the early stages of ALIGNMENT with the basic organizational needs identified in response to the Organizational Profile and other process items. (I)
50%, 55%, 60%, or 65%	• An EFFECTIVE, SYSTEMATIC APPROACH, responsive to the OVERALL QUESTIONS in the item, is evident. (A) • The APPROACH is well DEPLOYED, although DEPLOYMENT may vary in some areas or work units. (D) • Fact-based, SYSTEMATIC evaluation and improvement, and some examples of use of best practices, instances of INNOVATION, or sharing of refinements, are in place for improving the efficiency and EFFECTIVENESS of KEY PROCESSES. (L) • The APPROACH is ALIGNED with your overall organizational needs as identified in response to the Organizational Profile and other process items. (I)
70%, 75%, 80%, or 85%	• An EFFECTIVE, SYSTEMATIC APPROACH, responsive to MULTIPLE QUESTIONS in the item, is evident. (A) • The APPROACH is well DEPLOYED, with no significant gaps. (D) • Fact-based, SYSTEMATIC evaluation and improvement, adoption of best practices, managing for INNOVATION, and sharing of refinements are KEY tools for improving organizational efficiency and EFFECTIVENESS. (L) • The APPROACH is INTEGRATED with your current and future organizational needs as identified in response to the Organizational Profile and other process items. (I)
90%, 95%, or 100%	• An EFFECTIVE, SYSTEMATIC APPROACH, fully responsive to the MULTIPLE QUESTIONS in the item, is evident. (A) • The APPROACH is fully DEPLOYED without significant weaknesses or gaps in any areas or work units. (D) • Fact-based, SYSTEMATIC evaluation and improvement, development of best practices, achievement of INNOVATION, and sharing of refinements are KEY organization-wide tools for improving efficiency and EFFECTIVENESS. (L) • The APPROACH is well INTEGRATED with your current and future organizational needs as identified in response to the Organizational Profile and other process items. (I)

Terms in SMALL CAPS are defined in the Glossary of Key Terms (pages 46–53).

Results Scoring Guidelines (For Use with Category 7)

SCORE	DESCRIPTION
0% or 5%	• There are no organizational PERFORMANCE RESULTS, or the RESULTS reported are poor. (Le) • TREND data either are not reported or show mainly adverse TRENDS. (T) • Comparative information is not reported. (C) • RESULTS are not reported for any areas of importance to the accomplishment of your organization's MISSION. (I)
10%, 15%, 20%, or 25%	• A few organizational PERFORMANCE RESULTS are reported, responsive to the BASIC QUESTION in the item, and early good PERFORMANCE LEVELS are evident. (Le) • Some TREND data are reported, with some adverse TRENDS evident. (T) • Little or no comparative information is reported. (C) • RESULTS are reported for a few areas of importance to the accomplishment of your organization's MISSION. (I)
30%, 35%, 40%, or 45%	• Good organizational PERFORMANCE LEVELS are reported, responsive to the BASIC QUESTION in the item. (Le) • Some TREND data are reported, and most of the TRENDS presented are beneficial. (T) • Early stages of obtaining comparative information are evident. (C) • RESULTS are reported for many areas of importance to the accomplishment of your organization's MISSION. (I)
50%, 55%, 60%, or 65%	• Good organizational PERFORMANCE LEVELS are reported, responsive to the OVERALL QUESTIONS in the item. (Le) • Beneficial TRENDS are evident in areas of importance to the accomplishment of your organization's MISSION. (T) • Some current PERFORMANCE LEVELS have been evaluated against relevant comparisons and/or BENCHMARKS and show areas of good relative PERFORMANCE. (C) • Organizational PERFORMANCE RESULTS are reported for most KEY patient, other CUSTOMER, market, and PROCESS requirements. (I)
70%, 75%, 80%, or 85%	• Good-to-excellent organizational PERFORMANCE LEVELS are reported, responsive to MULTIPLE QUESTIONS in the item. (Le) • Beneficial TRENDS have been sustained over time in most areas of importance to the accomplishment of your organization's MISSION. (T) • Many to most TRENDS and current PERFORMANCE LEVELS have been evaluated against relevant comparisons and/or BENCHMARKS and show areas of leadership and very good relative PERFORMANCE. (C) • Organizational PERFORMANCE RESULTS are reported for most KEY patient, other CUSTOMER, market, PROCESS, and ACTION PLAN requirements. (I)
90%, 95%, or 100%	• Excellent organizational PERFORMANCE LEVELS are reported that are fully responsive to the MULTIPLE QUESTIONS in the item. (Le) • Beneficial TRENDS have been sustained over time in all areas of importance to the accomplishment of your organization's MISSION. (T) • Industry and BENCHMARK leadership is demonstrated in many areas. (C) • Organizational PERFORMANCE RESULTS and PROJECTIONS are reported for most KEY patient, other CUSTOMER, market, PROCESS, and ACTION PLAN requirements. (I)

Terms in SMALL CAPS are defined in the Glossary of Key Terms (pages 46–53).

From Fighting Fires to Innovation: An Analogy for Learning

Learning is an essential attribute of high-performing organizations. Effective, well-deployed organizational learning can help an organization improve from the early stages of reacting to problems to the highest levels of organization-wide improvement, refinement, and innovation.

1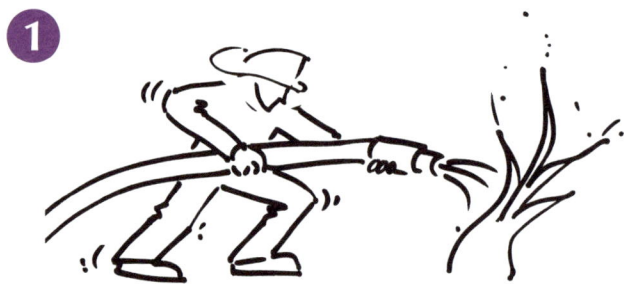

Reacting to the problem (0–5%)
Run with the hose and put out the fire.

2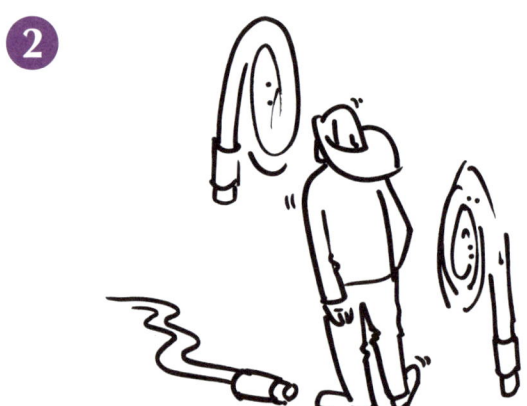

General improvement orientation (10–25%)
Install more fire hoses to get to the fires quickly and reduce their impact.

3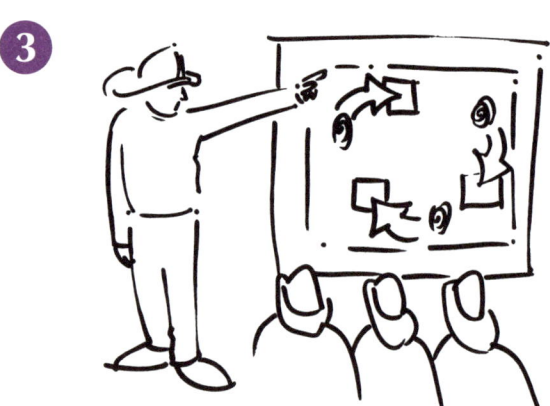

Systematic evaluation and improvement (30–45%)
Evaluate which locations are most susceptible to fire. Install heat sensors and sprinklers in those locations.

4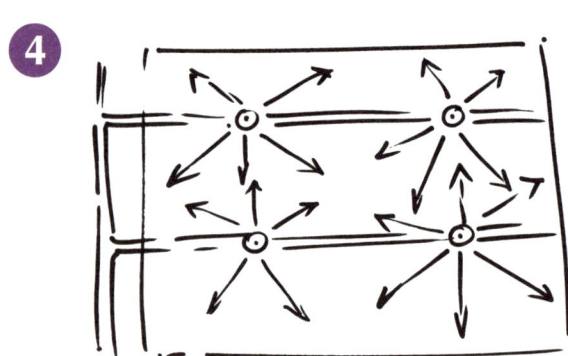

Learning and strategic improvement (50–65%)
Install systemwide heat sensors and a sprinkler system that is activated by the heat preceding fires.

5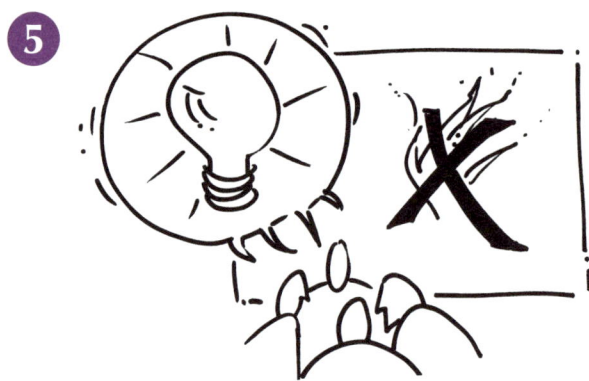

Organizational analysis and innovation (70–100%)
Use fireproof and fire-retardant materials. Replace combustible liquids with water-based liquids. Prevention is the primary approach for protection, with sensors and sprinklers as the secondary line of protection. This approach has been shared with all facilities and is practiced in all locations.

How to Respond to the Health Care Criteria

These guidelines explain how to respond most effectively to the questions in the 17 process and results Health Care Criteria items. This information is intended mainly for applicants for Baldrige-based awards, but it is also useful to organizations that are using the Health Care Criteria for self-assessment. See also the Scoring System, including the scoring guidelines (pages 32–33), which describes how to assess responses and determine your organization's performance accomplishments.

First Steps

1. Learn about the Baldrige framework.

Become familiar with the following sections, which provide a full orientation to the Baldrige framework:

- Health Care Criteria for Performance Excellence (pages 4–28)

- Scoring System (pages 29–34)

- Glossary of Key Terms (pages 46–53)

- Category and Item Commentary (https://www.nist.gov /baldrige/baldrige-criteria-commentary-health-care)

2. Understand how to read and respond to a Criteria item.

Review the Health Care Criteria for Performance Excellence Structure (page 2), which shows the types of items, the different parts of the items, and the role of each part. Pay particular attention to the multiple questions within the areas to address and the notes.

Some item questions include multiple parts. To respond fully, address all the questions, as missing information will be interpreted as a gap in your performance management system. Taken together, the multiple questions express the full meaning of the area to address. In responding, you may want to group responses to these questions in a way that is appropriate to your organization. You do not need to answer each question separately.

3. Review the scoring guidelines.

Consider both the Criteria and the scoring guidelines (pages 32–33) as you prepare your responses. In responding to the questions in the process items (categories 1–6), include information on the process evaluation factors in the scoring guidelines: the maturity of your approaches, the extent of their deployment, the extent of learning, and the extent of integration with other elements of your performance management system.

Similarly, in responding to the questions in the results items (category 7), include information on the results evaluation factors in the scoring guidelines: the actual performance levels, the significance of the results trends, relevant comparative data, integration with important elements of your performance management system, and the results of the improvement process. The "goodness" of your responses to the Criteria questions is determined through consideration of the evaluation dimensions (ADLI/LeTCI; see "Responding to Process Items" and "Responding to Results Items" below).

4. Understand the meaning of key terms.

Many terms in the Criteria and scoring guidelines have meanings that may differ somewhat from common meanings. When this is the case, the term is printed in SMALL CAPS and defined in the Glossary of Key Terms (pages 46–53). Understanding these terms can help you accurately self-assess your organization and communicate your processes and results to those reviewing your responses and planning your improvement efforts.

5. Start with the Organizational Profile.

The Organizational Profile (pages 4–6) is the most appropriate starting point. Whether you are using the Criteria as a leadership and management guide, or for self-assessment, writing an application, or reviewing either of these, the Organizational Profile helps you understand what is most relevant and important to your organization's business, mission, and performance.

Responding to Process Items

Although the Criteria focus on key organizational performance results, these results by themselves offer little *diagnostic* value. For example, if some results are poor or are improving at rates slower than your competitors' or comparable organizations' results, you need to understand why this is so and what you might do to accelerate improvement.

Your responses to process items (categories 1–6) permit you or those who are reviewing your responses to diagnose your organization's *most important* processes—the ones that contribute most to organizational performance improvement and result in key outcomes or performance results. This diagnosis and the quality of the feedback you receive depend heavily on the content and completeness of your responses. For this reason, respond to these items by providing information on your *key* processes. Guidelines for organizing and reviewing such information follow.

1. Understand the meaning of *how.*

In responding to questions in process items that begin with *how*, give information on your key processes with regard to approach, deployment, learning, and integration (ADLI; see the Scoring System, page 29). Responses lacking such information, or merely providing an example, are referred to in the scoring guidelines as *anecdotal information.*

Show that *approaches* are systematic. Systematic approaches are repeatable and use data and information to enable learning. In other words, approaches are systematic if they build in the opportunity for evaluation, improvement, innovation, and knowledge sharing, thereby enabling a gain in maturity.

Show *deployment.* In your responses, summarize how your approaches are implemented in different parts of your organization.

Show evidence of *learning.* Give evidence of evaluation and improvement cycles for processes, as well as adoption of best practices and innovations. Show that improvements are shared with other appropriate units of your organization to enable organizational learning.

Show *integration.* Integration is alignment and harmonization among processes, plans, measures, actions, and results. This harmonization greatly increases organizational effectiveness and efficiencies.

Showing alignment in the process items and tracking corresponding measures in the results items should improve organizational performance. In your responses, show alignment in four areas:

- In the Organizational Profile, make clear what is important to your organization.

- In Strategy (category 2), including the strategic objectives, action plans, and core competencies, highlight your organization's areas of greatest focus and describe how you deploy your strategic plan.

- In describing organizational-level analysis and review (item 4.1), show how you analyze and review performance information as a basis for setting priorities.

- In Strategy (category 2) and Operations (category 6), highlight the work systems and work processes that are key to your organization's overall performance.

2. Understand the meaning of *what.*

What questions set the context for showing alignment and integration in your performance management system. For example, when you identify key strategic objectives, your action plans, some performance measures, and some results in category 7 are expected to relate to those strategic objectives.

Two types of questions in process items begin with *what.* The first requests basic information on key processes and how they work. The second asks you to report key findings, plans, objectives, goals, or measures.

Responding to Results Items

1. Focus on your organization's most critical performance results.

Report results that cover the most important requirements for your organization's success, as highlighted in the Organizational Profile and in the Leadership, Strategy, Customers, Workforce, and Operations categories.

2. Report levels, trends, and comparisons, and show integration.

Report *performance levels* on a meaningful measurement scale.

Report *trends* to show the directions of results and rates of change in areas of importance. A minimum of three historical data points is generally needed to ascertain the beginnings of a trend. Trends represent historic and current performance, not projected (future) performance.

There is no minimum period for trend data; time intervals between data points should be meaningful for the measure(s) you report. Trends might span five or more years or less than one year, depending on what is meaningful. For important results, include new data even if trends are not yet well established. *Explain trends that show a significant beneficial or adverse change.*

Report *comparisons* to show how your results compare with those of other, appropriately selected organizations or benchmarks.

Show *integration* by including all results that are important to your organization, and segmenting them appropriately (e.g., by important patient, other customer, workforce, process, and service line groups, usually outlined in the Organizational Profile).

Responding Efficiently

1. Cross-reference when appropriate.

Ensure that each item response is as self-contained as possible and that responses to different items are mutually reinforcing. To accomplish this, refer to other responses rather than repeat information. In such cases, give key process information in the item requesting that information. For example, you would describe workforce development and learning systems in item 5.2. Discussions about workforce development and learning elsewhere in your application would then reference but not repeat details given in item 5.2.

2. Use a compact format.

To make the best use of space, use flowcharts, tables, and lists to present information concisely. Page limits for Baldrige Award and Baldrige-based award applications are designed to force your organization to consider what is most important in managing your enterprise and reporting your results.

3. Use graphs and tables.

You can report many results compactly by using graphs and tables. When you report results over time or compare them with others, "normalize" them (i.e., present them in a way—for example, as ratios—that takes size factors into account). For example, if the number of employees has varied over the period or if you are comparing your results to those of organizations differing in size, safety trends will be more meaningful if you report them as lost workdays per 100 employees rather than as total lost workdays.

The graph below shows one part of a possible response to item 7.1, Health Care and Process Results. In the Organizational Profile, the organization has identified use of beta-blockers with acute myocardial infarction (AMI) as a key requirement.

The graph illustrates a number of characteristics of clear and effective results reporting:

- Both axes and units of measure are clearly labeled.

- Levels and trends are reported for a key requirement—use of beta-blockers for AMI.

- Results are presented for several years.

- An arrow indicates that an upward trend is good for this measure.

- Appropriate comparisons are shown clearly.

- In a single graph, the organization shows that it tracks all three of its hospitals separately for beta-blocker use.

- The organization projects improved performance, including discontinuous or breakthrough improvement in 2021 relative to prior performance for hospital B. The text should explain this breakthrough change and might refer to critical learning from hospital A as the basis for the projected change.

Interpreting the graph with the scoring guidelines in mind would result in the following observations on the organization's performance and maturity level:

- The current overall organizational performance level is excellent. This conclusion is supported by the comparison with the best competitor and a national benchmark level.

- The overall organization shows beneficial improvement trends sustained over time.

- Hospital A is the current performance leader—showing sustained high performance and a slightly beneficial trend since 2017. Hospital B shows rapid improvement. Its performance is close to that of the best competitor but trails hospital A.

- Hospital C—identified in the text as a new acquisition—is having early problems with ensuring beta-blocker use but is projecting a turnaround. (The organization should briefly explain these problems.)

- The organization has projected improvements in beta-blocker use for all of its hospitals. Hospital C continues to lag behind the others; hospital A is projected to reach the benchmark level by 2021.

Figure 7.1-3 Beta-Blocker Use

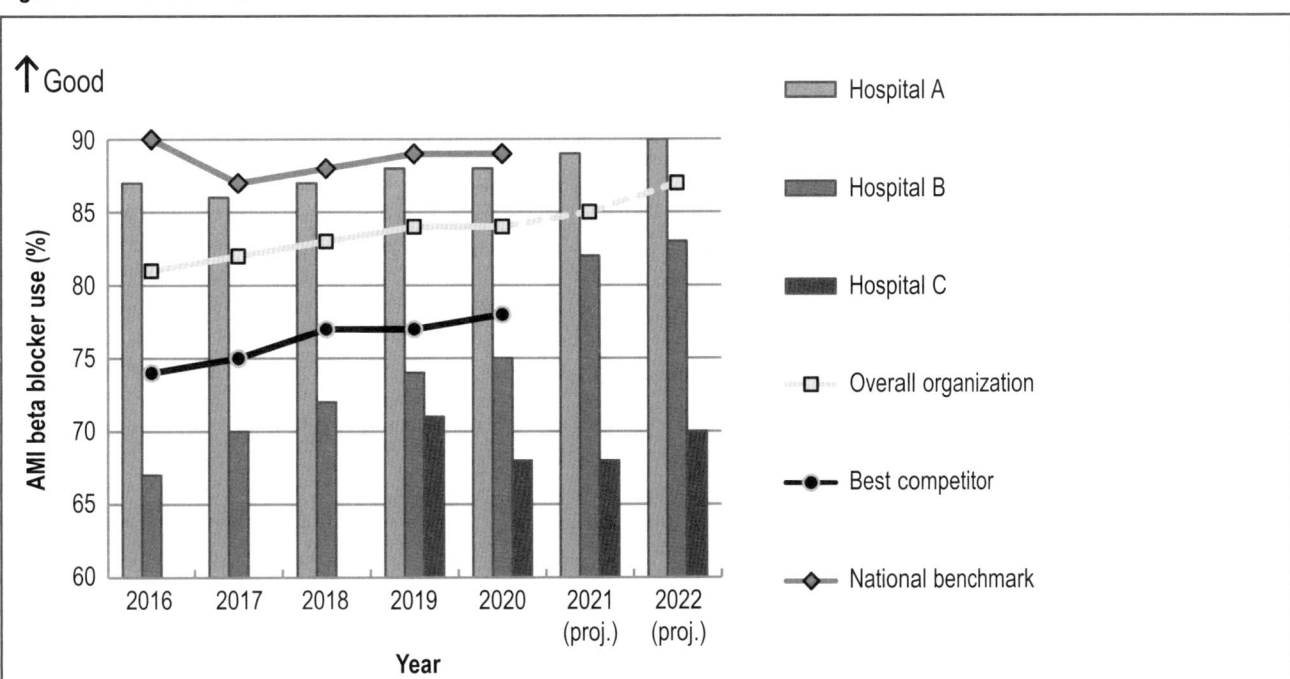

Core Values and Concepts

These beliefs and behaviors are embedded in high-performing organizations. They are the foundation for integrating key performance and operational requirements within a results-oriented framework that creates a basis for action, feedback, and ongoing success.

The Baldrige Health Care Criteria are built on the following set of interrelated core values and concepts:

- Systems perspective
- Visionary leadership
- Patient-focused excellence
- Valuing people
- Agility and resilience
- Organizational learning
- Focus on success and innovation
- Management by fact
- Societal contributions and community health
- Ethics and transparency
- Delivering value and results

Systems Perspective

A systems perspective means managing all the components of your organization as a unified whole to achieve your mission, ongoing success, and performance excellence. A systems perspective also means managing your organization within the context of an interconnected ecosystem of organizations that presents opportunities for new and possibly innovative relationships.

Successfully managing overall organizational performance requires realization of your organization as a system with interdependent operations. Organization-specific synthesis, alignment, and integration make the internal system successful. *Synthesis* means understanding your organization as a whole. It incorporates key organizational attributes, including your core competencies, strategic objectives, action plans, work systems, and workforce needs. *Alignment* means using key organizational linkages to ensure consistency of plans, processes, measures, and actions. *Integration* builds on alignment, so that the individual components of your performance management system operate in a fully interconnected, unified, and mutually beneficial manner to deliver anticipated results.

In addition, your organization exists within an organizational ecosystem—a network of organizations, including your partners, suppliers, collaborators, competitors, patients, other customers, communities, and other relevant organizations inside and outside the health care industry. Within this larger system, roles between organizations may be fluid as opportunities arise and needs change. For your ecosystem,

synthesis means understanding your organization as part of a larger whole. It incorporates the key attributes that you contribute to and need from your partners, collaborators, competitors, patients, other customers, communities, and other relevant organizations, including those not traditionally considered as collaborators.

These concepts are depicted in the Baldrige Health Care Criteria overview (page 1). When your organization takes a systems perspective, your senior leaders focus on strategic directions and on patients and other customers. Your senior leaders monitor, respond to, and manage performance based on your results. With a systems perspective, you use your measures, indicators, core competencies, and organizational knowledge to build your key strategies, link these strategies with your work systems and key processes, manage risk, and align your resources to improve your overall performance and your focus on patients, other customers, and stakeholders. The core values and concepts, the seven Health Care Criteria categories, and the scoring guidelines are the system's building blocks and integrating mechanism.

Visionary Leadership

Your organization's senior leaders should create a leadership system that includes both health care provider and administrative/operational leaders. This system should foster the integration and alignment of health care and business directions.

Your organization's senior leaders should set a vision for the organization, create a focus on patients and other customers, demonstrate clear and visible organizational values and ethics, and set high expectations for the workforce. The vision, values, and expectations should balance the needs of all your stakeholders. Your leaders should also ensure the creation of strategies, systems, and methods for building knowledge and capabilities, empowering the workforce, capitalizing on diversity, stimulating innovation, managing risk, ensuring resilience, requiring accountability, achieving performance excellence, and thereby ensuring ongoing organizational success.

The values and strategies leaders define should help guide all of your organization's activities and decisions. Senior leaders should inspire and encourage your entire workforce to contribute, to develop and learn, to be innovative, and to embrace meaningful change. Senior leaders should be responsible to your organization's governance body for their actions and performance, and the governance body should be responsible ultimately to all your stakeholders for your organization's and its senior leaders' ethics, actions, and performance.

Senior leaders should serve as role models through their ethical behavior and their personal involvement in planning, providing a supportive environment for innovation, communicating, coaching and motivating the workforce, developing future leaders, recognizing workforce members, promoting equity and inclusion, and reviewing organizational performance. Senior leaders should demonstrate authenticity and admit to their missteps and opportunities for improvement. As role models, they can reinforce ethics, values, and expectations while building leadership, commitment, and initiative throughout your organization.

Patient-Focused Excellence

Your patients and other customers are the ultimate judges of your performance and the quality of your health care services. Thus, your organization must consider all features and characteristics of patient care delivery (including those not directly related to medical, clinical, and health services), all modes of customer access and support, and all organizational values and behaviors that contribute value to your patients and other customers. Such behavior leads to patient acquisition, satisfaction, preference, trust, and loyalty; positive referrals; and, ultimately, your organization's ongoing success. Patient-focused excellence has both current and future components: understanding the desires of patients and other customers today and anticipating future desires and health care marketplace potential.

Many factors may influence value and satisfaction over the course of your patients' and other customers' experience with your organization. Primary among these factors is the degree of patient safety throughout the health care delivery process. Another factor is your management of patient and other customer relationships, which helps build trust, confidence, and loyalty. Additional factors include ease of access to care, the availability of clear information on likely health and functional status outcomes and on the cost of care, the responsiveness of health care providers and ancillary staff members, the opportunity for patients to participate in decisions about their health care, and the quality and availability of continuing care. This leads to the requirement for developing systems and processes to ensure that patients and family members are fully involved in the care team, educated so they fully understand their condition and the plan of care, and supported in making the medical decisions that are best for them.

Patient-focused excellence means much more than reducing errors, merely meeting accreditation specifications, or reducing complaints. Nevertheless, these factors contribute to your patients' and other customers' view of your organization and thus are also important parts of patient-focused excellence. In addition, your success in recovering from accidents, service errors, and mistakes; fostering equity and inclusion; adapting to disruptions; and safeguarding patient information is crucial for retaining patients and other customers and engaging them for the long term. Patient-focused excellence also involves increasing the efficiency and effectiveness of the services and care provided, and working to ensure that care is provided in the most appropriate setting.

A patient-focused organization addresses not only the health care service characteristics that meet basic patient and other customer requirements but also those unique features and characteristics that differentiate the organization from competitors. This differentiation may be based on an excellent patient experience, innovative health care service offerings or patient conveniences, combinations of offerings, price, customized offerings, multiple access and outward communication mechanisms, time to appointment, rapid response, your organization's societal contributions, or special relationships. These might include participation in alliances or collaborative, multilateral networks (ecosystems) of organizations that drive efficiency, effectiveness, and innovation.

A major long-term investment associated with health care excellence is investment in creating and sustaining an assessment system focused on health care outcomes. This entails becoming familiar with research findings and ongoing application of assessment methods. Patient-focused excellence is thus a strategic concept. It is directed toward patient and other customer retention and loyalty, referral of new patients, stronger brand recognition, market share gain, and growth. It demands constant sensitivity to changing and emerging patient, other customer, and market requirements and to the factors that drive customer engagement. It demands close attention to the voice of the customer. It demands anticipating changes in the marketplace. Therefore, patient-focused excellence demands a patient-focused culture and organizational agility.

Valuing People

An organization's success depends on an engaged workforce that benefits from meaningful work, clear organizational direction, the opportunity to learn, and accountability for performance. That workforce must also have a safe, trusting, and cooperative environment. The successful organization has a culture of equity and inclusion that capitalizes on the diverse backgrounds and characteristics, knowledge, skills, creativity, and motivation of its workforce, partners, collaborators, and patients. Promoting equity means ensuring that all patients and workforce members are treated fairly, and that all workforce members can reach their full potential. Inclusion refers to empowering participation and promoting a sense of belonging. The successful organization also values all people who have a stake in the organization, including patients, other customers, community members, stockholders, and other people affected by the organization's actions.

Valuing the people in your workforce means committing to their engagement, development, and well-being. Major challenges in valuing your workforce members include (1) demonstrating your leaders' commitment to their success; (2) providing motivation and recognition that go beyond the regular compensation system; (3) supporting work-life balance through flexible work practices tailored to varying workplace and life needs; (4) creating an inclusive, equitable environment for a diverse workforce; (5) offering development and progression within your organization; (6) providing support during disruptions and transitions; (7) sharing your organization's knowledge so that your workforce can better serve your patients and other customers and contribute to achieving your strategic objectives; (8) creating an environment that encourages intelligent risk taking to achieve innovation; and (9) developing a system of workforce and organizational accountability for performance. With increased remote work, an additional challenge is ensuring that a geographically dispersed workforce benefits from meaningful work, clear organizational direction, the opportunity to learn, and accountability for performance.

The success of your workforce members—including your leaders—depends on their having opportunities to learn. This learning includes preparing people for future organizational core competencies. On-the-job training offers a cost-effective way to cross-train and to link training more closely to your organization's capacity needs and priorities. Workforce members' learning includes building discipline knowledge and retraining to adjust to a changing health care environment, and enhancing knowledge of measurement systems that influence outcome assessments and clinical guidelines, decision trees, care bundles, or critical pathways. If your organization relies on volunteers, their personal development and learning are also important to consider.

To accomplish their overall goals, successful organizations build and value ecosystems of internal and external partnerships and collaborative, multilateral alliances. Internal partnerships might include cooperation among administrators, staff, physicians, and independent practitioners, as well as between labor and management. Forming internal partnerships might also involve creating network relationships among people across work units and locations, between physicians and other caregivers, or between employees and volunteers to improve flexibility, responsiveness, learning, and knowledge sharing, as well as to support the effective flow of patients through the health care system.

As health care services become more and more multidisciplinary, organizations may need new business models and ecosystems, including nontraditional partnerships with competitors or organizations outside the sector, alliances, consortia, and value networks.

Agility and Resilience

Success in today's ever-changing, competitive environment demands agility and organizational resilience. Agility requires a capacity for rapid change and for flexibility in operations. Organizational resilience is the ability to anticipate, prepare for, and recover from disasters, emergencies,

The Role of Core Values and Concepts

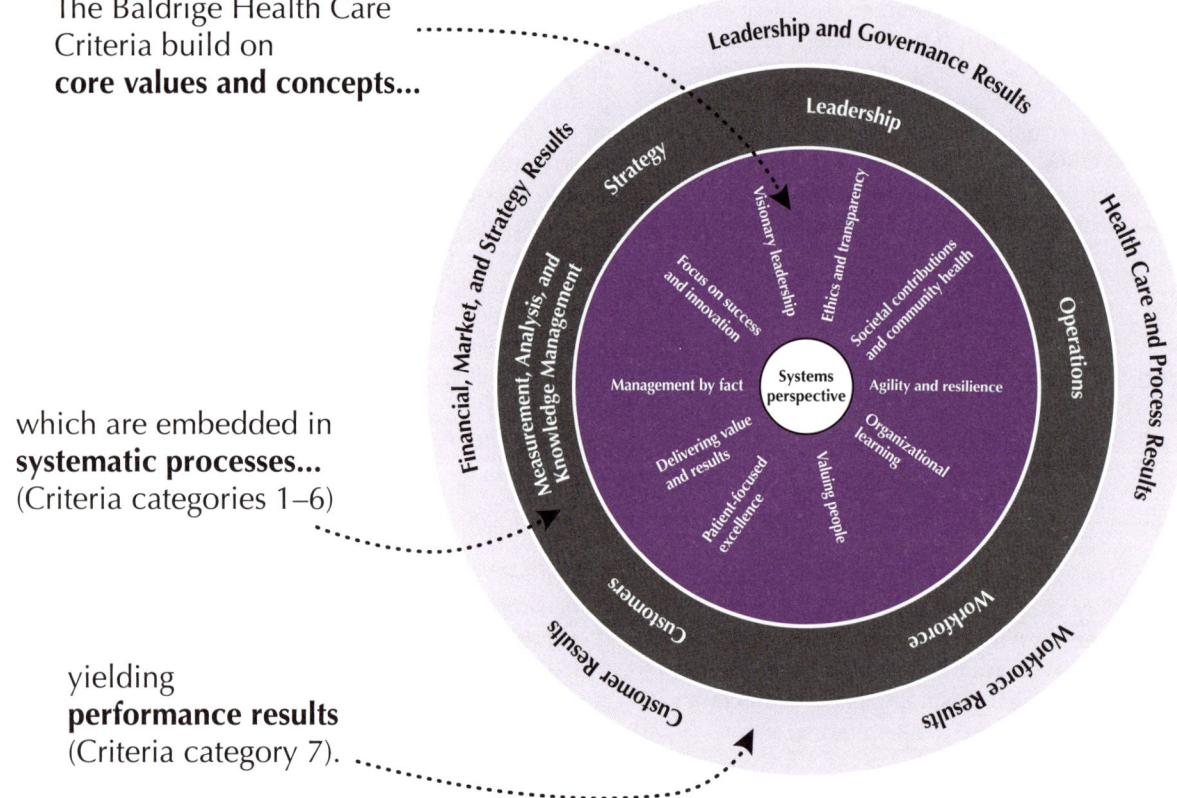

The Baldrige Health Care Criteria build on **core values and concepts...**

which are embedded in **systematic processes...** (Criteria categories 1–6)

yielding **performance results** (Criteria category 7).

and other disruptions, and—when disruptions occur—to protect and enhance workforce and customer engagement, supply-network and financial performance, organizational productivity, and community well-being. Resilience includes the agility to modify plans, processes, and relationships whenever circumstances warrant.

Health care organizations face ever-shorter cycles for introducing new or improved health care services, for faster and more flexible responses to patients and other customers, and for responding rapidly to new or emerging issues. Organizations must be capable of managing risk and making changes on an ever-shorter cycle time. Major improvements in response times often require new work systems; rapid decision making; reduced bureaucracy; the simplification of work processes; agile, efficient supplier and partner networks; effective, efficient communication with the workforce, partners, and suppliers; and the ability for rapid changeover from one process or one location to another.

All aspects of time performance are now more critical, and cycle time is a key process measure. Other important benefits can be derived from this focus on time; time improvements often drive simultaneous improvements or changes in your work systems, organization, quality, cost, supply-network integration, productivity, and ongoing success in a challenging economy. Today's health care environment places a heavy burden on organizations to ensure the timely design of health care delivery systems, disease prevention programs, health promotion programs, and effective and efficient diagnostic and treatment systems. Their design must value patients' individual needs and input, and include effective means of gauging the improvement of health status—for patients and populations or for communities. To meet the demands of rapidly changing markets, your organization needs to carry out stage-to-stage integration of activities from research or concept to implementation.

Disruptive events are occurring more frequently, triggered by economic upheaval or stress, major weather or health events, social or societal demands, or innovative technologies or product introductions. For an organization to be resilient, leaders must cultivate the agility to anticipate opportunities and threats, adapt strategy to changing circumstances, and have robust governance with a culture of trust. Organizations must embrace data-rich thought processes and equip their employees with ongoing learning of new skills.

Agility and resilience can also be achieved through your business ecosystem, in which collaborations, strategic partnerships, or alliances might offer complementary core competencies that allow rapid response to disruptions, entry into new markets or a basis for new health care services, referrals or shared facilities, or a rethinking of customer offerings in a larger context. Your ecosystem might also permit you to address common issues quickly by blending your organization's core competencies or leadership capabilities with other organizations' complementary strengths and capabilities, creating a new source of strategic

advantage. External partnerships might address sectorwide issues, such as the need for longitudinal care, equity of and access to care, and social determinants of health. The result may be broad, interdependent, agile ecosystems that include traditional partners and collaborators, as well as competitors, customers, communities, and organizations outside the health care industry.

Organizational Learning

Achieving the highest levels of organizational performance requires a well-executed approach to organizational learning that includes sharing knowledge via systematic processes. In today's demanding environment, a cross-trained and empowered workforce and effective management of up-to-date organizational knowledge are vital assets. Organizational learning includes continuous improvement of existing approaches; the adoption of best practices and innovations; and significant, discontinuous change or innovation, leading to new goals, approaches, health care services, and markets.

Learning needs to be embedded in the way your organization operates. This means that learning (1) is a regular part of daily work; (2) results in solving problems at their source (root cause); (3) is focused on building and sharing knowledge throughout your organization; and (4) is driven by opportunities to effect significant, meaningful change and to innovate. Sources for learning include employees', physicians', and volunteers' ideas; health care research findings; patients' and other customers' input; best-practice sharing; competitors' performance; and benchmarking. Your organizational ecosystem is another source of learning.

Organizational learning can result in (1) enhanced value to patients through new and improved services; (2) the development of new health care business opportunities; (3) the development of evidence-based approaches to medicine, new and improved processes, and new health care delivery models; (4) reduced errors, defects, waste, and related costs; (5) increased productivity and effectiveness in the use of all your resources; (6) enhanced performance in making societal contributions and building community health; and (7) greater agility in managing change and disruption.

Focus on Success and Innovation

Ensuring your organization's success now and in the future requires an understanding of the short- and longer-term factors that affect your organization and its environment. It also requires the ability to drive organizational innovation.

Sustained success requires managing uncertainty in the environment, as well as balancing some stakeholders' short-term demands with the need to invest in long-term success. The pursuit of sustained growth and performance leadership requires a strong future orientation and a willingness to make long-term commitments to key stakeholders—patients, their families, other customers, workforce, suppliers, partners, and community; the public; and employers, payors, and health profession students. It also requires the agility to modify plans, processes, and relationships whenever circumstances warrant.

Your organization's planning and resource allocation should anticipate many factors, such as changes in health care delivery models; changes in your supply network; resource availability; patients' and other customers' short- and long-term expectations; new business models and collaboration or partnering opportunities; potential crises, including events that disrupt economic and social conditions; technological developments; workforce capacity and capability needs; community and societal expectations and needs; your competitive marketplace; security and cybersecurity risks; evolving regulatory requirements; and strategic moves by competitors. Your strategic objectives and resource allocations need to accommodate these influences. A focus on success includes ensuring resilience; developing your leaders, workforce, and suppliers; accomplishing effective succession planning; and anticipating areas for societal contributions and concerns.

A focus on success also includes a focus on innovation—making meaningful change to improve health care services, programs, processes, operations, the health care delivery model, business models, or societal well-being, with the purpose of creating new value for stakeholders. Innovation should lead your organization to new dimensions of performance and success. Innovation may be present in organizations of all sizes, sectors, and maturity levels; in some cases, an organization's genesis is an innovation, with work systems and work processes developing as the organization matures.

Innovation is important for all aspects of your operations and all work systems and work processes. Innovation benefits from a supportive environment, a process for identifying strategic opportunities, and the pursuit of intelligent risks. Innovation and continuous incremental improvement are different, but complementary, concepts. Successful organizations use both approaches to improve performance. Your organization should be led and managed so that identifying strategic opportunities and taking intelligent risks become part of the learning culture. Innovation should be integrated into daily work and be supported by your performance improvement system. Systematic processes for identifying strategic opportunities should reach across your entire organization and should explore strategic alliances with complementary organizations and with organizations that have historically been outside your ecosystem.

Innovation may arise from adapting innovations in other industries to achieve a breakthrough. It builds on the accumulated knowledge of your organization and its people and the innovations of partners, collaborators, competitors, and other relevant organizations, including those outside the health care sector. It may involve collaboration among people who do not normally work together and are in different parts of the organization. This can lead to the maximizing of learning through shared information and the willingness to use concepts from outside the organization as idea generators. Therefore, the ability to rapidly disseminate and capitalize on new and accumulated knowledge is critical to driving organizational innovation and success.

Management by Fact

Management by fact requires you to measure and analyze your organization's performance, both inside the organization and in your competitive environment. Measurements should derive from organizational needs and strategy, and they should provide critical data and information about key processes, outputs, results, outcomes, and competitor and industry performance. Organizations need many types of data and information to effectively manage their performance. Data and information may come in many forms, such as numerical, graphical, or qualitative, and from many sources, including internal processes, surveys, and the Internet (including social media). Performance measurement should include measurement of health care outcomes; patient, other customer, service, and process performance; comparisons of operational, market, and competitive performance; supplier, workforce, partner, cost, and financial performance; governance and compliance results; and accomplishment of strategic objectives.

A major consideration in performance improvement and change management is the selection and use of performance measures or indicators. *The measures or indicators you select should best represent the factors that lead to improved health care outcomes; improved patient, other customer, operational, financial, and societal performance; and healthier communities. A comprehensive yet carefully culled set of measures or indicators tied to patient/other customer and organizational performance requirements provides a clear basis for aligning all processes with your organization's goals.* Measures and indicators support you in making decisions in a rapidly changing environment. By analyzing data from your tracking processes, you can evaluate the measures or indicators themselves and change them to better support your goals.

Analysis means extracting larger meaning from data and information to support evaluation, decision making, improvement, and innovation. It entails using data to determine trends, projections, and cause-and-effect relationships that might not otherwise be evident. Analysis supports a variety of purposes, such as planning, reviewing your overall performance, improving operations, comparing your performance with competitors' or with best-practice benchmarks, and managing change. To facilitate analysis, data may need to be aggregated from various sources. Data may also need to be segmented by, for example, markets, health care service lines, and workforce groups to gain deeper understanding.

Societal Contributions and Community Health

Your organization's leaders should stress contributions to the public, the consideration of societal well-being and benefit, and the need to foster improved community health. Leaders should be role models for your organization and its workforce in the protection of public health, safety, and the environment. This protection applies to any impact of your organization's operations. Also, your organization should emphasize resource conservation, recycling, and waste reduction at the source. Planning should anticipate adverse impacts from facilities management, as well as from distribution, transportation, use, and disposal of medical waste, radiation waste, chemicals, and biohazards. Effective planning should reduce or prevent problems; provide for a forthright response if problems occur; and make available the information and support needed to maintain public awareness, safety, and confidence.

Your organization should meet all local, state, and federal laws and regulatory requirements and should also treat these and related requirements as opportunities to excel beyond minimal compliance.

Considering societal well-being and benefit means leading and supporting—within the limits of your resources—the environmental, social, and economic systems in your organization's sphere of influence. Public health services and the support of the general health of the community are important societal responsibilities of health care organizations. Such leadership and support might include efforts to determine and address social determinants for health, such as by establishing free clinics or affordable health care programs, increasing public health awareness programs, or fostering neighborhood services for the elderly. It also might involve being a role model for addressing socially important issues, such as diversity, equity, and inclusion; practicing resource conservation; reducing your carbon footprint; performing community service and charity; improving health care industry practices; and sharing nonproprietary information. Increasingly, such societal contributions are a customer or stakeholder requirement.

For a role-model organization, leadership also entails influencing other organizations, private and public, to partner for these purposes. Managing societal contributions requires your organization to use appropriate measures and your leaders to assume responsibility for those measures.

Ethics and Transparency

Your organization should stress ethical behavior in all stakeholder transactions and interactions. Your organization's governance body should require highly ethical conduct and monitor all conduct accordingly. Ethical conduct should address both business and health care practices, such as nondiscriminatory patient treatment policies and the protection of patients' rights and privacy. Your senior leaders should be role models of ethical behavior and make their expectations of the workforce very clear.

Your organization's ethical principles are the foundation for your culture and values. They distinguish right from wrong. Clearly articulated ethical principles, along with your organizational values, empower your people to make effective decisions and may serve as boundary conditions for determining organizational norms and prohibitions.

Transparency is characterized by consistently candid and open communication, accountability, and the sharing of clear and accurate information by leadership and management. The benefits of transparency are manifold. Transparency is a key factor in workforce engagement and allows people to see why actions are being taken and how they can contribute. Transparency and accountability are also important in interactions with patients, customers, and other stakeholders, giving them a sense of involvement, engagement, and confidence in your organization.

Ethical behavior and transparency build trust in the organization and its leaders and engender a belief in the organization's fairness and integrity that is valued by all key stakeholders.

Delivering Value and Results

By delivering and balancing value for key stakeholders, your organization builds loyalty, contributes to growing the economy, and contributes to society. To meet the sometimes conflicting and changing aims that balancing value requires, your organizational strategy should explicitly include key stakeholder requirements. This will help ensure that plans and actions meet differing stakeholder needs and avoid adverse impacts on any stakeholders. A balanced composite of leading and lagging performance measures is an effective means to communicate short- and longer-term priorities, monitor actual performance, and provide a clear basis for improving results.

Your organization's performance measurements need to focus on key results. Results should be used to deliver and balance value for your key stakeholders—your patients and their families; payors; other customers; your workforce, suppliers, partners, and collaborators; health profession students; investors; the public; and the community. Thus, results need to be a composite of measures that include not just financial results but also health care and process results; patient, other customer, and workforce satisfaction and engagement results; and leadership, strategy, and societal performance.

Changes from the 2019–2020 Baldrige Excellence Framework

Revisions have one overarching purpose: for the framework and the Criteria to reflect the leading edge of validated leadership and performance practice while ensuring that they are as concise and user-friendly as possible.

For more than 30 years, the Criteria for Performance Excellence have evolved along with the drivers of organizational competitiveness and long-term success. Through this evolution, the Baldrige Excellence Framework offers today's organizations a nonprescriptive leadership and management guide that facilitates a systems approach to achieving excellence.

As the Baldrige framework and the Criteria evolve, they must balance two important considerations. On the one hand, the Criteria need to reflect a national standard for performance excellence, educating organizations in all aspects of establishing an integrated performance management system. On the other hand, the Criteria need to be accessible and user-friendly for a variety of organizations at varying levels of maturity.

To strike this balance, changes reflected in the *2021–2022 Baldrige Excellence Framework* focus on raising or strengthening organizations' awareness of the need for organizational resilience; the benefits of diversity, equity, and inclusion; and the ongoing digitization of nearly all aspects of organizational operations and management. Other changes clarify the role of innovation in organizational competitiveness and success, and expand the framework's focus on societal responsibility. Other changes throughout the Criteria clarify the intent of questions.

Resilience. Agility (a capacity for rapid change and for flexibility in operations) has long been a part of the Core Values and Concepts. The accelerating pace of change and the more frequent occurrence of disruptions—from economic upheaval or stress, major weather or health events, social or societal demands, or the introduction of innovative technologies or health care services—means that organizations must now focus on resilience. Resilience is the ability to anticipate, prepare for, and recover from disasters, emergencies, and other disruptions, and—when disruptions occur—to protect and enhance workforce, patient, and other customer engagement; supply-network and financial performance; organizational productivity; and community well-being. Resilience includes the agility to modify plans, processes, and relationships whenever circumstances warrant. The core value titled Agility has been broadened to Agility and Resilience, and the term "resilience" is defined in the Glossary of Key Terms. In the Criteria, organizational resilience is a focus of business continuity planning. It is also a consideration for leaders, in strategic planning, for work accomplishment, and in supply-network management.

Equity and inclusion. Expanding on the concept that the successful organization capitalizes on the diverse backgrounds and characteristics, knowledge, skills, creativity, and motivation of people, this revision of the Baldrige framework includes a stronger focus on equity and inclusion. The core values titled Patient-Focused Excellence, Valuing People, and Societal Contributions and Community Health now include this stronger focus, and equity and inclusion are now considerations for organizational culture and for patient, other customer, and workforce engagement, as well as in notes throughout the Criteria.

Digitization and the fourth industrial revolution. In today's digitally and data-enhanced economy, the use of data analytics, the Internet of Things, artificial intelligence, the adoption of cloud operations, large dataset-enabled business and process modeling, enhanced automation, and other "smart" technologies is accelerating rapidly. Although these tools may not affect all organizations currently or directly, they will most likely affect the competitive environment and new competitors. Notes on digitization and "big data" have been augmented throughout the Criteria. Questions on strategic planning and workforce change, as well as notes throughout the Criteria, now include these concepts, complementing the existing focus on incorporating new technology into health care service and process design.

Innovation. Since 2001, the Baldrige framework has emphasized the role of innovation in organizational success. This revision makes that relationship explicit by combining two previously separate core values into one, titled Focus on Success and Innovation. The Core Values and Concepts state that innovation may be present in organizations of all maturity levels; an innovation may even be the genesis of an organization. Revisions to the Scoring System, Process Scoring Guidelines, and definition of innovation in the Glossary of Key Terms reflect this clarification. In addition, the definition of innovation now includes the concept of making meaningful change to improve societal well-being.

Societal contributions. This concept has been present in the Baldrige framework since its inception in 1988 (as Public Responsibility), and changes since then have reflected the evolution of the role of societal contributions for successful organizations of all types. High-performing organizations see contributing to society as more than something they must do. Going above and beyond responsibilities in contributing to society can be a driver of patient, other customer, and workforce engagement, and a market differentiator. Employees, patients, other customers, and communities increasingly exhibit an interest in organizational social purpose and in how organizations contribute to society. Questions on societal contributions and strategy development, as well as notes throughout the Criteria, now include this strengthened focus.

The most significant changes to the Criteria items are summarized as follows.

Category 1: Leadership

Item 1.1, Senior Leadership, now includes questions about creating an organizational culture that fosters patient, other customer, and workforce equity and inclusion, and about cultivating organizational resilience.

In item 1.2, questions now ask how you incorporate, rather than consider, societal well-being and benefit as part of your strategy and daily operations.

Category 2: Strategy

In item 2.1, Strategy Development, questions now ask how your strategic planning process addresses resilience and how you consider relevant technological changes and innovations in your planning.

Category 3: Customers

Item 3.2, Customer Engagement, now asks how your patient and other customer experience processes ensure fair treatment for all customers.

Category 5: Workforce

In item 5.1, questions now ask how you prepare your workforce for changes in workplaces and technology, and how you organize and manage your workforce to reinforce organizational resilience and agility.

In item 5.2, Workforce Engagement, a new area to address asks how you ensure that your performance management, performance development, and career development approaches promote equity and inclusion, and an existing question has been expanded to ask how you ensure that your organizational culture promotes equity and inclusion.

Category 6: Operations

In item 6.1, Work Processes, the fourth area to address is now called Management of Opportunities for Innovation. A note explains that your process for pursuing opportunities

for innovation should capitalize on strategic opportunities identified as intelligent risks, as well as intelligent risks arising from performance reviews, knowledge management, and other sources of potential innovations.

In item 6.2, the third area to address is now titled Safety, Business Continuity, and Resilience. The questions clarify that your safety systems should consider your workforce, your patients, and other people in your workplace. The item also includes questions on how you ensure that your organization can anticipate, prepare for, and recover from disasters, emergencies, and other disruptions.

Category 7: Results

Item 7.1 now asks specifically for patient safety results. Item 7.4, Leadership and Governance Results, now asks for your results for leaders' communication and engagement to cultivate innovation and intelligent risk taking.

Scoring System

The explanation of the learning evaluation factor clarifies that learning comprises (1) the refinement of approaches through cycles of evaluation and improvement, (2) the adoption of best practices and innovations, and (3) the sharing of refinements and innovations. The Process Scoring Guidelines now specifically refer to these components. Like Baldrige scoring in general, scoring for the learning factor is holistic: the organization's achievement level in one component is not a "gate" blocking a score in a particular range.

Core Values

The concept of agility, formerly paired with organizational learning, now forms part of the core value titled Agility and Resilience. The core value titled Focus on Success and Innovation pairs two formerly separate, but complementary, concepts.

Glossary of Key Terms

The Glossary of Key Terms now includes a definition of the term resilience. The definition of innovation now reflects the clarifications described above. One term, cycle time, has been deleted, as the definition used in the Criteria reflects the definition that is in common use.

Glossary of Key Terms

The terms below are those in SMALL CAPS *in the Baldrige Health Care Criteria for Performance Excellence and scoring guidelines. Each term is followed by a definition in boldface. The rest of the first paragraph elaborates on this definition. The paragraphs that follow provide examples, descriptive information, or key linkages to other information about the Baldrige framework.*

ACTION PLANS. Specific actions that your organization takes to reach its strategic objectives. These plans specify the resources committed to and the time horizons for accomplishing the plans. Action plan development is the critical stage in planning when you make strategic objectives and goals specific so that you can effectively deploy them throughout the organization in an understandable way. In the Criteria, deploying action plans includes creating aligned measures for all affected departments and work units. Deployment might also require specialized training for some workforce members or recruitment of personnel.

For example, a strategic objective for a health care system in an area with an active business alliance focusing on cost and quality of care might be to become the low-cost provider. Action plans could entail designing efficient processes to optimize the length of hospital stays, reduce rework resulting from patient injuries and treatment errors, analyze resource and asset use, and analyze the most commonly encountered diagnosis-related groups with a focus on prevention in those areas. To deploy the action plans, the system might train department and work-unit caregivers in setting priorities based on costs and benefits. Organizational-level analysis and review would likely emphasize process efficiency, cost per patient, and health care quality.

See also STRATEGIC OBJECTIVES.

ALIGNMENT. A state of consistency among plans, processes, information, resource decisions, workforce capability and capacity, actions, results, and analyses that support key organization-wide goals. Effective alignment requires a common understanding of purposes and goals. It also requires the use of complementary measures and information for planning, tracking, analysis, and improvement at three levels: the organizational level, the key process level, and the departmental or work-unit level.

See also INTEGRATION.

ANALYSIS. The examination of facts and data to provide a basis for effective decisions. Analysis often involves determining cause-effect relationships. Overall organizational analysis guides you in managing work systems and work processes toward achieving key organizational results and attaining strategic objectives.

Although individual facts and data are important, they do not usually provide an effective basis for acting or setting priorities.

Effective actions depend on an understanding of relationships, which is derived from the analysis of facts and data.

ANECDOTAL. In a response to a Health Care Criteria item, information that lacks specific methods; measures; deployment mechanisms; and evaluation, improvement, and learning factors. Anecdotal information frequently consists of examples and describes individual activities rather than systematic processes. For example, in an anecdotal response to how senior leaders deploy performance expectations, you might describe a specific occasion when a senior leader visited all of your organization's facilities. On the other hand, in describing a systematic process, you might include the methods all senior leaders use to communicate performance expectations regularly to all locations and workforce members, the measures leaders use to assess the effectiveness of the methods, and the tools and techniques you use to evaluate and improve the methods.

See also SYSTEMATIC.

APPROACH. The methods your organization uses to carry out its processes. Besides the methods themselves, approach refers to the appropriateness of the methods to the item questions and your organization's operating environment, as well as how effectively your organization uses those methods.

Approach is one of the factors considered in evaluating process items. For further description, see the Scoring System (pages 29–34).

BASIC QUESTION. The most central concept of a Health Care Criteria item, as presented in the item title question. For an illustration, see Health Care Criteria for Performance Excellence Structure (page 2).

BENCHMARKS. Processes and results that represent the best practices and best performance for similar activities, inside or outside your organization's industry. Organizations engage in benchmarking to understand the current dimensions of world-class performance and to achieve discontinuous (nonincremental) or "breakthrough" improvement.

Benchmarks are one form of comparative data. Other forms include health care data collected by a third party (e.g., CMS, accrediting organizations, and commercial organizations), data on competitors' and other organizations' performance obtained from sharing or from external reference databases, comparisons with similar organizations that are in the same geographic area or that provide similar health care services, and information from the open literature (e.g., outcomes of research studies and practice guidelines).

CAPABILITY, WORKFORCE. See WORKFORCE CAPABILITY.

CAPACITY, WORKFORCE. See WORKFORCE CAPACITY.

COLLABORATORS. Organizations or individuals who cooperate with your organization to support a particular activity or event or who cooperate intermittently when their short-term goals are aligned with or are the same as yours. Typically, collaborations do not involve formal agreements or arrangements.

See also PARTNERS.

CORE COMPETENCIES. Your organization's areas of greatest expertise; those strategically important, possibly specialized capabilities that are central to fulfilling your mission or that provide an advantage in your marketplace or service environment. Core competencies are frequently challenging for competitors or suppliers and partners to imitate, and they may provide an ongoing competitive advantage or create opportunities in your business ecosystem. The absence of a needed core competency may result in a significant strategic challenge or disadvantage for your organization in the marketplace.

Core competencies may involve technological expertise, unique service offerings, a marketplace niche, or business acumen in a particular area (e.g., start-ups).

CUSTOMER. An actual or potential user of your organization's health care services. Customers include the direct users of your health care services (patients), as well as those who pay for your services, such as patients' families, insurers, and other third-party payors. The Baldrige framework addresses customers broadly, referencing your current and future patients and other customers, as well as your competitors' patients and other customers.

Patient-focused excellence is a Baldrige core value embedded in the beliefs and behaviors of high-performing organizations. Patient focus impacts and should be a factor in integrating your organization's strategic directions, work systems and work processes, and organizational performance results.

See also STAKEHOLDERS for the relationship between customers and others affected by your health care services.

CUSTOMER ENGAGEMENT. Your patients' and other customers' investment in or commitment to your brand and health care service offerings. It is based on your ongoing ability to serve their needs and build relationships so that they will continue using your services. Characteristics of engaged customers include retention, brand loyalty, willingness to make an effort to obtain—and to continue to obtain—health care services from you, and willingness to actively advocate for and recommend your brand and service offerings.

DEPLOYMENT. The extent to which your organization applies an approach in addressing the questions in a Health Care Criteria item. Evaluation of deployment considers how broadly and deeply the approach is applied in relevant work units throughout your organization.

Deployment is one of the factors considered in evaluating process items. For further description, see the Scoring System (pages 29–34).

DIVERSITY. Personal differences among workforce members that enrich the work environment and are representative of your hiring and patient communities. These differences address many variables, such as race, religion, color, gender, national origin, disability, sexual orientation, age and generation, education, geographic origin, and skill characteristics, as well as ideas, thinking, academic disciplines, and perspectives.

The Health Care Criteria refer to valuing and benefiting from the diversity of your workforce hiring and patient communities. Capitalizing on both in building your workforce increases your opportunities for high performance; patient, other customer, workforce, and community satisfaction; and patient, other customer, and workforce engagement.

EFFECTIVE. How well a process or a measure addresses its intended purpose. Determining effectiveness requires (1) evaluating how well the process is aligned with the organization's needs and how well it is deployed, or (2) evaluating the outcome of the measure as an indicator of process or service performance.

EMPOWERMENT. Giving people the authority and responsibility to make decisions and take actions. When people are empowered, decisions are made closest to patients and other customers (the front line), where work-related knowledge and understanding reside.

The purpose of empowering people is to enable them to satisfy patients and other customers on first contact, improve processes and increase productivity, and improve your organization's health care and other performance results, as well as to encourage collaboration. An empowered workforce requires information to make appropriate decisions; thus, your organization must provide that information in a timely and useful way.

ENGAGEMENT, CUSTOMER. See CUSTOMER ENGAGEMENT.

ENGAGEMENT, WORKFORCE. See WORKFORCE ENGAGEMENT.

ETHICAL BEHAVIOR. The actions your organization takes to ensure that all its decisions, actions, and stakeholder interactions conform to its moral and professional principles of conduct. These principles should support all applicable laws and regulations and are the foundation for your organization's culture and values. They distinguish right from wrong.

Senior leaders should be role models for these principles of behavior. The principles apply to all people involved in your organization, from temporary workforce members to members of the board of directors. These principles benefit from regular communication and reinforcement. Senior leaders have the responsibility for the alignment of your organization's mission and vision with its ethical principles. Ethical behavior encompasses interactions with all stakeholders, including your workforce, patients and their family members, insurers, payors, other customers, other partners, suppliers, and local community.

Well-designed and clearly articulated ethical principles empower people to make effective decisions with great confidence. In some organizations, ethical principles also serve as boundary conditions restricting behavior that otherwise could have adverse impacts on your organization and/or society.

See also the core value, Ethics and Transparency (page 43).

EXCELLENCE. See PERFORMANCE EXCELLENCE.

GOALS. Future conditions or performance levels that your organization intends or desires to attain. Goals can be both short and longer term. They are ends that guide actions. Quantitative goals, frequently referred to as targets, include a numerical point or range. Targets might be desired performance based on comparative or competitive data. Stretch goals are goals for desired major, discontinuous (nonincremental) or "breakthrough" improvements, usually in areas most critical to your organization's future success.

Goals can serve many purposes, including

- clarifying strategic objectives and action plans to indicate how you will measure success,
- fostering teamwork by focusing on a common end,
- encouraging out-of-the-box thinking (innovation) to achieve a stretch goal, and
- providing a basis for measuring and accelerating progress.

See also PERFORMANCE PROJECTIONS.

GOVERNANCE. The system of management and controls exercised in the stewardship of your organization. Governance includes the responsibilities of your organization's owners/shareholders, board of directors, and senior leaders (administrative/operational and health care). Corporate or organizational charters, bylaws, and policies document the rights and responsibilities of each of the parties and describe how they will direct and control your organization to ensure (1) accountability to owners/shareholders and other stakeholders, (2) transparency of operations, and (3) fair treatment of all stakeholders. Governance processes may include the approval of strategic direction, the monitoring and evaluation of the CEO's performance, the establishment of executive compensation and benefits, succession planning, financial and other fiduciary auditing, risk management, disclosure, and shareholder reporting. Ensuring effective governance is important to stakeholders' and the larger society's trust and to organizational effectiveness.

HEALTH CARE SERVICES. All services delivered by your organization that involve professional clinical/medical judgment, including those delivered to patients and to the community. Health care services also include services that are not considered clinical or medical, such as admissions, food services, and billing.

HIGH PERFORMANCE. Ever-higher levels of overall organizational and individual performance, including quality, productivity, innovation rate, and cycle time. High performance results in improved service and value for patients, other customers, and other stakeholders.

Approaches to high performance vary in their form, their function, and the incentive systems used. High performance stems from and enhances workforce engagement. It involves cooperation between the administration/management and the workforce, which may involve workforce bargaining units; cooperation among work units, often involving teams; empowerment of your people, including personal accountability; and workforce input into planning. It may involve learning and building individual and organizational skills; learning from other organizations; creating flexible job design and work assignments; maintaining a flattened organizational structure, where decision making is decentralized and decisions are made closest to patients and other customers (the front line); and effectively using performance measures, including comparisons. Many organizations encourage high performance with monetary and nonmonetary incentives based on factors such as organizational performance, team and individual contributions, and skill building. Also, approaches to high performance usually seek to align your organization's structure, core competencies, work, jobs, workforce development, and incentives.

HOW. The systems and processes that your organization uses to achieve its mission requirements. In responding to "how" questions in Health Care Criteria categories 1–6, you should include information on approach (methods and measures), deployment, learning, and integration.

INDICATORS. See MEASURES AND INDICATORS.

INNOVATION. Making meaningful change to improve health care services, processes, the organization, or societal well-being and create new value for stakeholders. Innovation involves adopting an idea, process, technology, service, or business model that is either new or new to its proposed application. The outcome of innovation is a discontinuous or "breakthrough" improvement in results, services, processes, or societal well-being. Innovation benefits from a supportive environment, a process for identifying strategic opportunities, and a willingness to pursue intelligent risks.

Successful organizational innovation also entails knowledge sharing, a decision to implement, implementation, evaluation, and learning. Although innovation is often associated with health care research and technological innovation, it is applicable to all key organizational processes that can benefit from change through innovation, whether breakthrough improvement or a change in approach or outputs. Innovation may be present in organizations of all sizes, sectors, and maturity levels; in some cases, an organization's genesis is an innovative idea, process, technology, service, or change in organizational structure or business model.

See also INTELLIGENT RISKS and STRATEGIC OPPORTUNITIES.

INTEGRATION. The harmonization of plans, processes, information, resource decisions, workforce capability and capacity, actions, results, and analyses to support key organization-wide goals. Effective integration goes beyond alignment and is achieved when the individual components of an organizational performance management system operate as a fully interconnected unit.

Integration is one of the factors considered in evaluating both process and results items. For further description, see the Scoring System (pages 29–34).

See also ALIGNMENT.

INTELLIGENT RISKS. Opportunities for which the potential gain outweighs the potential harm or loss to your organization's future success if you do not explore them. Taking intelligent risks requires a tolerance for failure and an expectation that innovation is not achieved by initiating only successful endeavors. At the outset, organizations must invest in potential successes while realizing that some will lead to failure.

The degree of risk that is intelligent to take will vary by the pace and level of threat and opportunity in the health care sector. In a rapidly changing environment with constant introductions of new health care services, processes, or business models, there is an obvious need to invest more resources in intelligent risks than in a stable environment. In the latter, organizations must monitor and explore growth potential and change but, most likely, with a less significant commitment of resources.

See also STRATEGIC OPPORTUNITIES.

KEY. Major or most important; critical to achieving your intended outcome. The Health Care Criteria, for example, refer to key challenges, plans, work processes, and measures—those that are most important to your organization's success. They are the essential elements for pursuing or monitoring a desired outcome. Key is generally defined as around the most significant five (e.g., around five key challenges).

KNOWLEDGE ASSETS. Your organization's accumulated intellectual resources; the knowledge possessed by your organization and its workforce in the form of information, ideas, learning, understanding, memory, insights, cognitive and technical skills, and capabilities. These knowledge assets reside in your workforce, software, patents, databases, documents, guides, and policies and procedures. Knowledge assets also reside within patients, other customers, suppliers, and partners.

Knowledge assets are the know-how that your organization has available to use, invest, and grow. Building and managing knowledge assets are key components of creating value for your stakeholders and sustaining a competitive advantage.

LEADERSHIP SYSTEM. The way leadership is exercised, formally and informally, throughout your organization; the basis for key decisions and the way they are made, communicated, and carried out. A leadership system includes structures and mechanisms for making decisions; ensuring two-way communication; selecting and developing leaders and managers; and reinforcing values, ethical behavior, directions, and performance expectations. In health care organizations with separate administrative/operational and health care provider leadership, the system includes both sets of leaders and the relationship between them.

An effective leadership system respects workforce members' and other stakeholders' capabilities and requirements, and it sets high expectations for performance and performance improvement. It builds loyalties and teamwork based on your organization's vision and values and the pursuit of shared goals. It encourages and supports initiative, innovation, and appropriate risk taking; subordinates organizational structure to purpose and function; and avoids chains of command that require long decision paths. An effective leadership system includes mechanisms for leaders to conduct self-examination, receive feedback, and improve.

LEARNING. New knowledge or skills acquired through evaluation, study, experience, and innovation. The Baldrige framework refers to two distinct kinds of learning: organizational learning and learning by the people in your workforce. Organizational learning is achieved through research and development, evaluation and improvement cycles, ideas and input from the workforce and stakeholders, the sharing of best practices, and benchmarking. Workforce learning is achieved through education, training, and developmental opportunities that further individual growth.

To be effective, learning should be embedded in the way your organization operates. Learning contributes to a competitive advantage and ongoing success for your organization and workforce.

For further description of organizational and personal learning, see the related core values and concepts: Valuing People and Organizational Learning (pages 39, 40).

Learning is one of the factors considered in evaluating process items. For further description, see the Scoring System (pages 29–34).

LEVELS. Numerical information that places or positions your organization's results and performance on a meaningful measurement scale. Performance levels permit evaluation relative to past performance, projections, goals, and appropriate comparisons.

MEASURES AND INDICATORS. Numerical information that quantifies the input, output, and performance dimensions of processes, programs, projects, services, and the overall organization (outcomes). Measures and indicators might be simple (derived from one measurement) or composite.

The Health Care Criteria do not distinguish between measures and indicators. However, some users of these terms prefer "indicator" (1) when the measurement relates to performance but does not measure it directly (e.g., the number of complaints is an indicator but not a direct measure of dissatisfaction), and (2) when the measurement is a predictor ("leading indicator") of some more significant performance (e.g., increased patient satisfaction might be a leading indicator of retention of health maintenance organization members).

MISSION. Your organization's overall function. The mission answers the question, "What is your organization attempting to accomplish?" The mission might define patients, other customers or markets served, distinctive or core competencies, or technologies used.

MULTIPLE QUESTIONS. The details of a Health Care Criteria item, as expressed in the individual questions under each lettered area to address. The first question in a set of multiple questions expresses the most important one in that group. The questions that follow expand on or supplement that question. For an illustration, see Health Care Criteria for Performance Excellence Structure (page 2).

Even high-performing, high-scoring users of the Baldrige framework are not likely to be able to address all the multiple questions with equal capability or success.

OVERALL QUESTIONS. The most important features of a Health Care Criteria item, as elaborated in the first question (the leading question in boldface) in each paragraph under each lettered area to address. For an illustration, see Health Care Criteria for Performance Excellence Structure (page 2).

PARTNERS. Key organizations or individuals who are working in concert with your organization to achieve a common goal or improve performance. Typically, partnerships are formal arrangements for a specific aim or purpose, such as to achieve a strategic objective or deliver a specific health care service.

Formal partnerships usually last for an extended period and involve a clear understanding of the partners' individual and mutual roles and benefits.

See also COLLABORATORS.

PERFORMANCE. Outputs and their outcomes obtained from health care services, processes, patients, and other customers that permit you to evaluate and compare your organization's results to performance projections, standards, past results, goals, and other organizations' results. Performance can be expressed in nonfinancial and financial terms.

The Health Care Criteria address four types of performance: (1) health care process and outcome, (2) patient- and other customer-focused, (3) operational, and (4) financial and marketplace.

Health care process and outcome performance is performance relative to measures and indicators of characteristics of health care service delivery that are important to patients and other customers. Examples include hospital readmission rates, mortality and morbidity rates, measures of patient harm associated with the health care system, and length of hospital stays, as well as measures of functional status, out-of-hospital treatment of chronic conditions, culturally sensitive care, and patient compliance and adherence. Health care performance might be measured at the organizational level, the diagnosis-related-group level, or the patient segment level.

Patient- and other customer-focused performance is performance relative to measures and indicators of patients' and other customers' perceptions, reactions, and behaviors. Examples include patient and other customer retention, complaints, and survey results.

Operational performance is workforce, leadership, and organizational performance (including ethical and legal compliance) relative to measures and indicators of effectiveness, efficiency, and accountability. Examples include cycle time, productivity, waste reduction, workforce turnover, workforce cross-training rates, accreditation, regulatory compliance, fiscal accountability, strategy accomplishment, community involvement, and contributions to community health. Operational performance might be measured at the work-unit, key work process, and organizational levels.

Financial and marketplace performance is performance relative to measures of cost, revenue, and market position, including asset utilization, asset growth, and market share. Examples include returns on investments, value added per employee, bond ratings, debt-to-equity ratio, returns on assets, operating margins, performance to budget, the amount in reserve funds, days cash on hand, other profitability and liquidity measures, and market gains.

PERFORMANCE EXCELLENCE. An integrated approach to organizational performance management that results in (1) delivery of ever-improving value to patients, other customers, and stakeholders, contributing to improved health care quality and ongoing organizational success; (2) improvement of your organization's overall effectiveness and capabilities; and (3) learning for the organization and for people in the workforce. The Baldrige Organizational Profile, Health Care Criteria, core values and concepts, and scoring guidelines provide a framework and assessment tool for understanding your organization's strengths and opportunities for improvement and, thus, for guiding your planning toward achieving higher performance and striving for excellence.

PERFORMANCE PROJECTIONS. Estimates of your organization's future performance. Projections should be based on an understanding of past performance, rates of improvement, and assumptions about future internal changes and innovations, as well as assumptions about changes in the external environment that result in internal changes. Thus, performance projections can serve as a key tool in managing your operations and in developing and implementing your strategy.

Performance projections state your *expected* future performance. Goals state your *desired* future performance. Performance projections for your competitors or similar organizations may indicate challenges facing your organization and areas where breakthrough performance or innovation is needed. In areas where your organization intends to achieve breakthrough performance or innovation, your performance projections and your goals may overlap.

See also GOALS.

PROCESS. Linked activities with the purpose of producing a service for a customer (user) within or outside your organization. Generally, processes involve combinations of people, machines, tools, techniques, materials, and improvements in a defined series of steps or actions. Processes rarely operate in isolation and must be considered in relation to other processes that impact them. In some situations, processes might require adherence to a specific sequence of steps, with documentation (sometimes formal) of procedures and requirements, including well-defined measurement and control steps.

In the delivery of services, particularly those that directly involve patients and other customers, process is used more generally to spell out what delivering that service entails, possibly including a preferred or expected sequence. If a sequence is critical, the process needs to include information that helps customers understand and follow the sequence. Such service processes also require guidance for service providers on handling contingencies related to customers' possible actions or behaviors.

In knowledge work, such as strategic planning, research, development, and analysis, process does not necessarily imply formal sequences of steps. Rather, it implies general understandings of competent performance in such areas as timing, options to include, evaluation, and reporting. Sequences might arise as part of these understandings.

Process is one of the two dimensions evaluated in a Baldrige-based assessment. This evaluation is based on four factors: approach, deployment, learning, and integration. For further description, see the Scoring System (pages 29–34).

PRODUCTIVITY. Measures of the efficiency of resource use.

Although the term is often applied to single factors, such as the workforce (labor productivity), machines, materials, energy, and capital, the concept also applies to the total resources used in producing outputs. Using an aggregate measure of overall productivity allows you to determine whether the net effect of overall changes in a process— possibly involving resource trade-offs—is beneficial.

PROJECTIONS, PERFORMANCE. See PERFORMANCE PROJECTIONS.

RESILIENCE. An organization's ability to (1) anticipate, prepare for, and recover from disasters, emergencies, and other disruptions, and (2) protect and enhance workforce and customer engagement, supply-network and financial performance, organizational productivity, and community well-being when disruptions occur. Organizational resilience requires agility throughout the organization.

Beyond the ability to "bounce back" to a prior state when a disruption occurs, resilience means having a plan in place that allows your organization to continue operating as needed during disruptions. To achieve resilience, leaders must cultivate the agility to respond quickly to both opportunities and threats, adapt strategy to changing circumstances, and have robust governance with a culture of trust. Organizations must adopt an ecosystem mindset, embrace data-rich thought processes, and equip their employees with ongoing learning of new skills.

RESULTS. Outputs and outcomes achieved by your organization. Results are evaluated based on current performance; performance relative to appropriate comparisons; the rate, breadth, and importance of performance improvements; and the relationship of results measures to key organizational performance requirements.

Results are one of the two dimensions evaluated in a Baldrige-based assessment. This evaluation is based on four factors: levels, trends, comparisons, and integration. For further description, see the Scoring System (pages 29–34).

SEGMENT. One part of your organization's patient, other customer, market, health care service offering, or workforce base. Segments typically have common characteristics that allow logical groupings. In Health Care Criteria results items, segmentation refers to disaggregating results data in a way that allows for meaningful analysis of your organization's performance. It is up to each organization to determine the factors that it uses to segment its patients, other customers, markets, services, and workforce.

Understanding segments is critical to identifying the distinct needs and expectations of different patient, other customer, market, and workforce groups and to tailoring health care service offerings to meet their needs and expectations. For example, you might segment your market based on service volume, geography, or technologies employed. You might segment your workforce based on geography, skills, needs, specialties, work assignments, or job classifications.

SENIOR LEADERS. Your organization's senior management group or team. In many organizations, this consists of the head of the organization and his or her direct reports. In health care organizations with separate administrative/operational and health care provider leadership, "senior leaders" refers to both sets of leaders.

STAKEHOLDERS. All groups that are or might be affected by your organization's actions and success. Key stakeholders might include customers, the community, employers, health care providers, patient advocacy groups, departments of health, students, the workforce, partners, collaborators, governing boards, stockholders, donors, suppliers, taxpayers, regulatory bodies, policy makers, funders, and local and professional communities.

See also CUSTOMER.

STRATEGIC ADVANTAGES. Those marketplace benefits that exert a decisive influence on your organization's likelihood of future success. These advantages are frequently sources of current and future competitive success relative to other providers of similar health care services. Strategic advantages generally arise from either or both of two sources: (1) core competencies, which focus on building and expanding on your organization's internal capabilities, and (2) strategically important external resources, which your organization shapes and leverages through key external relationships and partnerships.

When an organization realizes both sources of strategic advantage, it can amplify its unique internal capabilities by capitalizing on complementary capabilities in other organizations.

See STRATEGIC CHALLENGES and STRATEGIC OBJECTIVES for the relationship among strategic advantages, strategic challenges, and the strategic objectives your organization articulates to address its challenges and advantages.

STRATEGIC CHALLENGES. Those pressures that exert a decisive influence on your organization's likelihood of future success. These challenges are frequently driven by your organization's anticipated and/or competitive position in the future relative to other providers of similar health care services. While not exclusively so, strategic challenges are generally externally driven. However, in responding to externally driven strategic challenges, your organization may face internal strategic challenges.

External strategic challenges may relate to patient, other customer, or market needs or expectations; health care service or technological changes; or financial, societal, and other risks or needs. Internal strategic challenges may relate to capabilities or human and other resources.

See STRATEGIC ADVANTAGES and STRATEGIC OBJECTIVES for the relationship among strategic challenges, strategic advantages, and the strategic objectives your organization articulates to address its challenges and advantages.

STRATEGIC OBJECTIVES. The aims or responses that your organization articulates to address major change or improvement, competitiveness or social issues, and health care advantages. Strategic objectives are generally focused both externally and internally and relate to significant patient, other customer, market, health care service, or technological opportunities and challenges (strategic challenges). Broadly stated, they are what your organization

must achieve to remain or become competitive and ensure its long-term success. Strategic objectives set your organization's longer-term directions and guide resource allocation and redistribution.

See ACTION PLANS for the relationship between strategic objectives and action plans and for an example of each.

STRATEGIC OPPORTUNITIES. Prospects for new or changed services, processes, business models (including strategic alliances), or markets. They arise from outside-the-box thinking, brainstorming, capitalizing on serendipity, research and innovation processes, nonlinear extrapolation of current conditions, and other approaches to imagining a different future.

The generation of ideas that lead to strategic opportunities benefits from an environment that encourages nondirected, free thought. Choosing which strategic opportunities to pursue involves consideration of relative risk, financial and otherwise, and then making intelligent choices (intelligent risks).

See also INTELLIGENT RISKS.

SYSTEMATIC. Well-ordered, repeatable, and exhibiting the use of data and information so that learning is possible. Approaches are systematic if they build in the opportunity for evaluation, improvement, and sharing, thereby permitting a gain in maturity. To see the term in use, refer to the Process Scoring Guidelines (page 32).

TRENDS. Numerical information that shows the direction and rate of change of your organization's results or the consistency of its performance over time. Trends show your organization's performance in a time sequence.

Ascertaining a trend generally requires a minimum of three historical (not projected) data points. Defining a statistically valid trend requires more data points. The cycle time of the process being measured determines the time between the data points for establishing a trend. Shorter cycle times demand more frequent measurement, while longer cycle times might require longer periods for a meaningful trend.

Examples of trends called for by the Health Care Criteria and scoring guidelines include data on health care outcomes and other health care service performance; results for patient, other customer, and workforce satisfaction and dissatisfaction; financial performance; marketplace performance; and operational performance, such as cycle time and productivity.

VALUE. The perceived worth of a program, service, process, asset, or function relative to its cost and possible alternatives.

Organizations frequently use value considerations to determine the benefits of various options relative to their costs, such as the value of various health care service combinations to patients and other customers. Your organization needs to understand what different stakeholder groups value and then deliver value to each group. This frequently requires balancing value among customers and other stakeholders, such as your workforce and the community.

VALUES. The guiding principles and behaviors that embody how your organization and its people are expected to operate. Values influence and reinforce your organization's desired culture. They support and guide the decisions made by every workforce member, helping your organization accomplish its mission and attain its vision appropriately. Examples of values include demonstrating integrity and fairness in all interactions, exceeding patients' and other customers' expectations, valuing individuals and diversity, protecting the environment, and striving for performance excellence every day.

VISION. Your organization's desired future state. The vision describes where your organization is headed, what it intends to be, or how it wishes to be perceived in the future.

VOICE OF THE CUSTOMER. Your process for capturing patient- and other customer-related information. Voice-of-the-customer processes are intended to be proactive and continuously innovative to capture stated, unstated, and anticipated patient and other customer requirements, expectations, and desires. The goal is to achieve customer engagement. Listening to the voice of the customer might include gathering and integrating various types of patient and other customer data, such as survey data, focus group findings, social media data and commentary, and complaint data, that affect patients' and other customers' relationship and engagement decisions.

WORK PROCESSES. Your organization's most important internal value-creation processes. They might include health care service design, production, and delivery; patient support; supply-network management; business; and support processes. They are the processes that involve the majority of your organization's workforce and produce patient, other customer, and stakeholder value.

Your key work processes are always accomplished by your workforce. They frequently relate to your core competencies, the factors that determine your success relative to competitors and organizations offering similar health care services, and the factors your senior leaders consider important for business growth. In contrast, projects are unique work processes intended to produce an outcome and then go out of existence.

WORK SYSTEMS. The coordinated combination of internal work processes and external resources that you need to develop and produce health care services, deliver them to your patients, and succeed in your market. Within your work systems, internal work processes are those that involve your workforce. External resources may include processes performed by your key suppliers, partners, contractors, and collaborators, as well as other components of your supply network needed to produce and deliver your health care services and carry out your business and support processes. These internal work processes and external resources function together to accomplish your organization's work.

Decisions about work systems are strategic, as you must decide whether to use internal processes or external resources for maximum efficiency and sustainability in your marketplace. These decisions involve protecting intellectual property, capitalizing on core competencies, and mitigating risk. The decisions you make have implications for your organizational structure, people, work processes, and equipment/technology.

WORKFORCE. All people actively supervised by your organization and involved in accomplishing your organization's work, including paid employees (e.g., permanent, part-time, temporary, on-site, and remote employees, as well as contract employees supervised by your organization), resident physicians, independent practitioners not paid by the organization (e.g., physicians, physician assistants, nurse practitioners, acupuncturists, and nutritionists), health care students (e.g., medical, nursing, and ancillary), and volunteers, as appropriate. Your workforce includes team leaders, supervisors, and managers at all levels.

WORKFORCE CAPABILITY. Your organization's ability to accomplish its work processes through its people's knowledge, skills, abilities, and competencies.

Capability may include the ability to build and sustain relationships with patients, other customers, and the community; to innovate and transition to new technologies; to develop new health care services and work processes; and to meet changing health care, market, and regulatory demands.

WORKFORCE CAPACITY. Your organization's ability to ensure sufficient staffing levels to accomplish its work processes and deliver your health care services to patients and other customers, including the ability to meet varying demand levels.

WORKFORCE ENGAGEMENT. The extent of workforce members' emotional and intellectual commitment to accomplishing your organization's work, mission, and vision. Organizations with high levels of workforce engagement are often characterized by high-performance work environments in which people are motivated to do their utmost for their patients' and other customers' benefit and the organization's success.

In general, workforce members feel engaged when they find personal meaning and motivation in their work and receive interpersonal and workplace support. An engaged workforce benefits from trusting relationships, a safe and cooperative environment, good communication and information flow, empowerment, and accountability for performance. Key factors contributing to engagement include training and career development, effective recognition and reward systems, equal opportunity and fair treatment, and family-friendliness. Workforce engagement also depends on building and sustaining relationships between your administrative/operational leadership and independent practitioners.

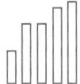

Index of Key Terms

*Page numbers in **boldface** indicate definitions in the Glossary of Key Terms (pages 46–53).*

G

Glossary of Key Terms, 46–53
goals, ii, iv, 8, 10, 19, 28, 29, 30, 31, 36, 40, 41, 42, 46, 47, **48**, 49, 50, 51
governance, 1, 3, 4, 7, 8, 9, 16, 25, 27, 28, 38, 40, 41, 42, 43, 45, **48**, 51

H

Health Care Criteria for Performance Excellence, 4–28
  items and point values, 3
  overview and structure, 1–2
health care outcomes, 6, 11, 17, 22, 25, 39, 40, 42, 50, 52
health care services, 4, 5, 6, 8, 10, 11, 12, 13, 14, 15, 17, 22, 23, 24, 25, 26, 30, 39, 40, 41, 42, 44, 47, **48**, 49, 50, 51, 52, 53
  design of, 10, 11, 22, 41, 44, 53
  improvement of, 22, 42, 48
  performance of, 13, 22, 25, 39, 50
  requirements for, 22, 29
high performance, ii, iii, 1, 7, 18, 19, 20, 37, 38, 44, 47, **48**, 50, 53
how (meaning of), 36, **48**
How to Respond to the Health Care Criteria, 35–37
How to Use the Baldrige Excellence Framework, v–vi

I

improvement
  breakthrough, 37, 42, 46, 48, 49, 51
  continuous, 16, 41, 42
  cycles of, iv, 29, 36, 45, 49
  of health care services and processes, 22, 42, 48
  opportunities for, ii, vi, 20, 29, 36, 39, 50, 52
  of performance, ii, v, vi, 1, 3, 6, 7, 16, 22, 23, 25, 29, 35, 36, 37, 38, 42, 47, 49, 50, 51
  tools for, iii, v, 6, 46
inclusion, iii, 7, 8, 11, 19, 39, 42, 44, 45
indicators. *See* measures and indicators of performance
information technology, iii, 18, 24
innovation, ii, iii, iv, v, vi, 5, 6, 7, 8, 10, 12, 13, 16, 17, 18, 21, 22, 23, 25, 26, 27, 29, 31, 32, 34, 36, 38, 39, 40, 41, 42, 44, 45, **48–49**, 51, 52, 53
  focus on success and (core value), ii, 38, 40, 41–42, 44, 45

integration (evaluation factor), iv, 1, 6, 29, 30, 31, 32, 33, 35, 36, 38, 48, **49**, 51
intelligent risks, iii, 7, 8, 10, 20, 22, 23, 27, 28, 40, 42, 45, 48, **49**, 52
items (Criteria), 2, 3

K

key (meaning of), **49**
knowledge, organizational, 10, 18, 22, 25, 38, 40, 41, 42, 49
knowledge assets, 16, 18, **49**
knowledge management, ii, iii, 1, 3, 12, 16, 17, 18, 23, 40, 45

L

leaders. *See* senior leaders
leadership, visionary (core value), ii, 38–39, 40
Leadership (category 1), ii, 1, 3, 5, 7–9, 25, 36, 40, 45
leadership system, v, 4, 5, 7, 8, 38, **49**
learning (evaluation factor), iv, vi, 6, 7, 12, 18, 29, 30, 31, 34, 35, 36, 37, 41, 45, 46, 48, **49**, 52
  organizational (core value), ii, 7, 18, 30, 31, 34, 36, 38, 40, 41, 42, 45, 49, 50
learning and development, workforce, 12, 20, 21, 36, 40, 41, 42, 48, 49, 50, 51
legal, regulatory, and accreditation compliance, iii, 8, 9, 42, 43, 50
LeTCI (levels, trends, comparisons, integration). *See* Scoring System and individual terms
levels (evaluation factor), iv, 29, 30, 33, 35, 36, 37, **49**, 51

M

management by fact (core value), ii, 38, 40, 42
Measurement, Analysis, and Knowledge Management (category 4), ii, 1, 3, 12, 16–18, 25, 40
measures and indicators (of performance), 8, 9, 12, 16, 17, 19, 20, 22, 25, 26, 27, 28, 29, 30, 31, 36, 38, 42, 43, 46, 48, 49, **50**, 51
mission, ii, 4, 5, 7, 9, 21, 33, 35, 38, 47, 48, **50**, 53
multiple (item) questions, 2, 32, 33, 35, **50**

O

Operations (category 6), ii, 1, 3, 9, 12, 19, 22–24, 25, 27, 36, 40, 45
opportunities for improvement, ii, vi, 20, 29, 36, 39, 50, 52
organizational learning, ii, 7, 18, 30, 31, 34, 36, 38, 40, 41, 42, 45, 49, 50
  as core value, ii, 38, 40, 41, 45
Organizational Profile (preface), iii, v, vi, 1, 2, 3, 4–6, 23, 25, 29, 30, 32, 35, 36, 37, 50
overall (item) questions, 2, 32, 33, **50**

P

partners, iii, 5, 7, 9, 10, 11, 12, 16, 18, 24, 26, 27, 38, 39, 40, 41, 42, 43, 47, 48, 49, **50**, 52, 53
patient. *See* patients and other customers
patient-focused excellence (core value), ii, 38, 39, 44, 47
patient safety, iii, 7, 8, 11, 20, 24, 25, 39, 45
patients and other customers, ii, iii, 4, 5, 7, 8, 9, 10, 11, 12, 13–14, 15, 17, 18, 19, 20, 21, 22, 23, 24, 25, 26, 27, 28, 29, 30, 33, 36, 38, 39, 40, 41, 42, 43, 44, 45, 46, 47, 48, 49, 50, 51, 52, 53
  dissatisfaction of, 14, 26, 50, 52
  engagement of, iii, 3, 7, 10, 13, 14, 26, 39, 41, 43, 44, 45, **47**, 51, 53
  groups (segments), 4, 5, 11, 13, 14, 25, 26, 27, 28, 36, 50, **51**
  listening to, iii, 13, 26, 53. *See also* voice of the customer
  loyalty of, iii, 13, 39, 43, 47
  relationships with, 13, 14, 26, 39, 47, 53
  requirements and expectations of, 4, 5, 11, 12, 13, 14, 19, 22, 23, 24, 25, 29, 30, 33, 39, 42, 43, 53
  retention of, 14, 39, 47, 50
  satisfaction of, 14, 15, 20, 23, 26, 39, 43, 47, 50, 52
  support of, 4, 5, 13, 14, 39, 53
performance, **50**
  customer-focused, 25, 26, 42, 50
  financial, market, and strategy, 25, 28, 41, 42, 50, 52
  health care process and outcome, 22, 23, 25, 42, 47, 50, 52

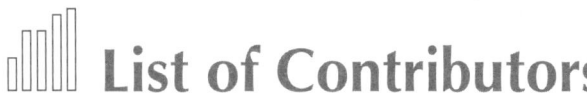

List of Contributors

The Baldrige Program thanks the following groups and individuals for contributing to the development of the 2021–2022 Baldrige Excellence Framework.

Alliance for Performance Excellence
Susan Allred
Deborah Ameen
Deborah Baehser
Mike Belter
Charles Bens
Board of Examiners of the Malcolm Baldrige
   National Quality Award
Board of Overseers of the Malcolm Baldrige
   National Quality Award
Glenn Bodinson
Dean Bondhus
Stephen Bonk
Scott Burgmeyer
Stan Butkus
Mara Bryant
Kathleen Carrothers
Dan Castle
Bonnie Charland
Mary Beth Corace
Bill Craddock
Catherine Craver
Glenn Crotty
Patricia Curtis
Bridget Dewees
Margaret Dospiljulian
Grace Duffy
Mark Erath
Joel Ettinger
Lindel Fields
Donald Fisher
Eric Fletcher
Jan Garfield
Linda Parker Gates
Kelly Gilhooly
Kathy Goerdt
Brenda Grant
Kevin Grayson

Pat Griffith
Paul Grizzell
Glenn Hamamura
G. F. Robert Hanke, Jr.
Marcia Harrington
Denise Haynes
Harry Hertz
Deanna Herwald
Margot Hoffman
Zoe Irvin
John Jasinski
Kathy Jenson
Jan Johnson
Kevin Johnson
Nancy Jokovich
Judges Panel of the Malcolm Baldrige
   National Quality Award
Beth Katzenberg
Kay Kendall
Heather Kenney
Marci Kenney
Marsha Kessler
Noureen Khan
Laura Kinney
Lori Kirkland
Miriam Kmetzo
Peter LaBonte
Les Lacy
Pat Lapekas
Brian Lassiter
Alice Lewis
Joe Marchese
Geri Markley
Debra McBride
James McCorvey
Mac McGuire
Kevin McManus
Anil Mengharajani

Liz Menzer
Brian Miller
Emily Miller
Sunil Mithas
John Molenda
Brigitta Mueller
Joe Muzikowski
Suresh Nirody
Larry Owen
S. Padmanabhan
Theron Post
Robert Rainer
Michael Reames
Bruce Requa
Glendali Rodriguez
Rob Rouzer
Brent Ruben
Terri Runyan
Doug Serrano
Denise Shields
Patricia Skriba
Tedd Snyder
Vicki Spagnol
Dennis Stambaugh
JoAnn Sternke
Tammie Strobel
Craig Thompson
John Van Gorkum
John Vinyard
Polly Walker
Brook Ward
Bob Warren
Meridith Wentz
Kevin Wilkinson
Sonja Wulff
Marlene Yanovsky
Mark Young
James Youngquist

Baldrige Performance Excellence Program

Created by Congress in 1987, the Baldrige Program is managed by the National Institute of Standards and Technology (NIST), an agency of the U.S. Department of Commerce. This unique public-private partnership is dedicated to helping organizations improve their performance and succeed in the global marketplace. The program administers the Presidential Malcolm Baldrige National Quality Award. In collaboration with the greater Baldrige community, we address critical national needs through

- a systems approach to achieving organizational excellence;

- organizational self-assessment tools and analysis of organizational strengths and opportunities for improvement by a team of trained experts;

- training, executive education, conferences, and workshops on proven best management practices and on using the Baldrige Excellence Framework to improve; and

- Baldrige-based approaches to cybersecurity risk management and community excellence.

Foundation for the Malcolm Baldrige National Quality Award

The mission of the Baldrige Foundation is to ensure the long-term financial growth and viability of the Baldrige Performance Excellence Program and to support organizational performance excellence in the United States and throughout the world. To learn more about the Baldrige Foundation and Institute for Performance Excellence, see www.baldrigefoundation.org or www.baldrigeinstitute.org.

Alliance for Performance Excellence

The Alliance (www.baldrigealliance.org) is a national network of Baldrige-based organizations and supporting members with a mission to grow performance excellence in support of a thriving Baldrige community. Members contribute nearly 300,000 volunteer hours and more than $30 million per year in tools, resources, and expertise to assist organizations on their journeys to excellence. This includes annually evaluating and recognizing over 1,000 organizations that use the Baldrige Excellence Framework and serving as the feeder system for the national Baldrige Award.

ASQ

ASQ (asq.org) assists in administering the award program under contract to NIST. ASQ is the leading membership association to help quality professionals achieve their career goals and drive excellence through quality in their organizations and industries. ASQ provides expertise, knowledge, networks, and solutions to a global membership of individuals spanning more than 130 countries. ASQ was founded in 1946 and is headquartered in Milwaukee, Wisconsin, USA.

For more information:

www.nist.gov/baldrige | 301.975.2036 | baldrige@nist.gov

The Malcolm Baldrige National Quality Award

www.nist.gov/baldrige/baldrige-award

The Malcolm Baldrige National Quality Award, created by Public Law 100-107 in 1987, is the highest level of national recognition for performance excellence that a U.S. organization can receive. The award promotes

- awareness of performance excellence as an increasingly important element in U.S. competitiveness and

- the sharing of successful performance strategies and information on the benefits of using these strategies.

The President of the United States traditionally presents the award. A 22-karat, gold-plated medallion bears the name of the award and "The Quest for Excellence" on one side and the Presidential Seal on the other.

Organizations apply for the award in one of six eligibility categories: manufacturing, service, small business, education, health care, and nonprofit. Up to 18 awards may be given annually across the six categories.

The Quest for Excellence® Conference

Official conference of the Malcolm Baldrige National Quality Award

www.nist.gov/baldrige/qe

April 12–15, 2021
April 3–6, 2022
April 2–5, 2023

Each year at The Quest for Excellence Conference, Baldrige Award recipients share their exceptional performance practices with leaders of business, education, health care, and nonprofit organizations and inspire attendees to apply the insights they gain within their own organizations.

Plan to attend and learn about the recipients' best management practices, participate in educational presentations on the Baldrige Excellence Framework, and network with Baldrige Award recipients and other attendees.

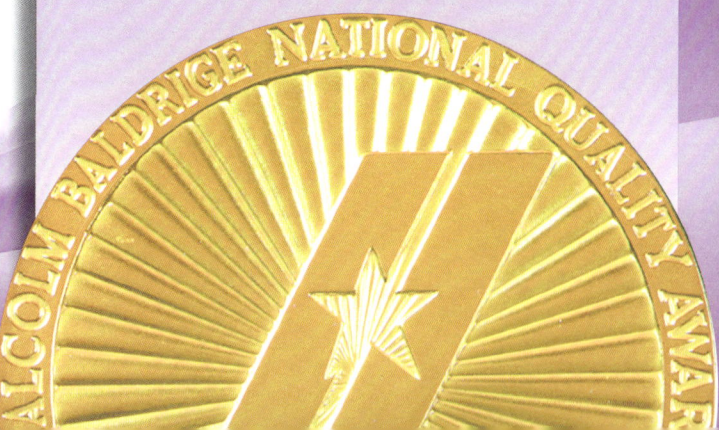

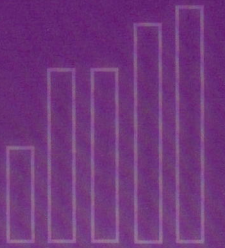

The ratio of the Baldrige Program's benefits for the U.S. economy to its costs is estimated at **820 to 1**.

121 Baldrige Award **winners** serve as national role models.

2010–2020 award applicants represent **676,535 jobs**, 5,001 work sites, over $189 billion in revenue/budgets, and about 614 million customers served.

248 Baldrige examiners volunteered roughly **$5.6 million** in services in 2020.

Baldrige-based programs annually evaluate and recognize more than **1,000 organizations** that use the Baldrige Excellence Framework.

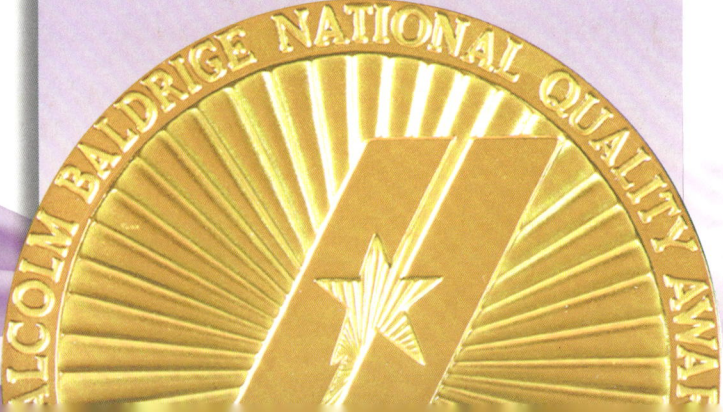

What People Are Saying

[Baldrige has] helped us create discipline around our processes, improved our financial performance, and improved our focus on key quality metrics.

Kyle Bennett
President and CEO
Memorial Hospital and Health Care Center
Jasper, IN
Baldrige Award recipient

Baldrige is a proven means of making your organization great for the people it serves and those who work for you. The framework supports long-term sustainability and leads to innovation.

Jayne Pope
CEO
Hill Country Memorial
Fredericksburg, TX
Baldrige Award recipient

CONNECT WITH BALDRIGE
@BaldrigeProgram #Baldrige

NIST
National Institute of
Standards and Technology
U.S. Department of Commerce

FSC MIX Paper from responsible sources FSC® C101537
www.fsc.org

$30.00
ISBN 978-0-9980827-7-6
53000>

T1661

9 780998 082776